AF379857

Springer

Tokyo
Berlin
Heidelberg
New York
Barcelona
Hong Kong
London
Milan
Paris
Singapore

K. Okita (Ed.)

Progress in Hepatocellular Carcinoma Treatment

With 32 Figures

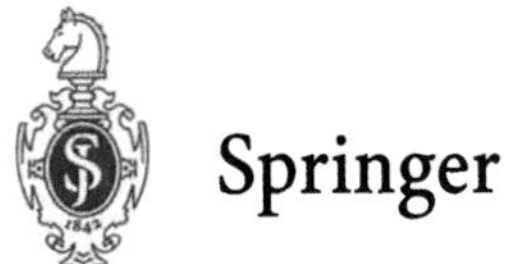

Springer

Kiwamu Okita, M.D., Ph.D.
Professor and Chairman
First Department of Internal Medicine
Yamaguchi University School of Medicine
1144 Kogushi, Ube, Yamaguchi 755-8505, Japan

ISBN 4-431-70257-1 Springer-Verlag Tokyo Berlin Heidelberg New York

Printed on acid-free paper

Typesetting: Best-set Typesetter Ltd., Hong Kong

SPIN: 10728634

Preface

According to a recent report from the Japanese Ministry of Health and Welfare, the mortality rate for hepatocellular carcinoma (HCC) is more than 30 per 100 000 population. In addition, epidemiologists predict an increase in this figure by the year 2015, because of the rather high incidence of chronic liver diseases caused by HCV. The same situation has been observed in other Asian countries.

It seems that HCC is likely to be an endemic disease, because of the higher prevalence of chronic hepatitis and liver cirrhosis caused by HBV, HCV, and/or aflatoxins in Asian and African countries. We also note that an interesting paper appeared in a recent issue of the *New England Journal of Medicine* describing the increase in younger HCC patients in the United States as compared with past decades. At present, silent hepatitis C infection is now smoldering in 4 million mostly unsuspecting Americans. Those carriers will be candidates for chronic liver disease, which is a predisposing factor for the development of HCC. In Europe there are an estimated 5 million carriers. Accordingly, it is important to do all we can to reduce the prevalence of HCC not only in African and Asian countries, but also in the United States and Europe.

With this perspective, last year the Japanese Society for Hepatology, in cooperation with the Ministry of Health and Welfare, initiated a national campaign to fight HCC. To begin with, we prepared a white paper and a pamphlet for public distribution, to provide accurate, up to date information on HCC in Japan. Against the background of our society's efforts, the Organizing Committee of the Yamaguchi Symposium on Liver Disease chose "Progress in HCC Treatment" as the main topic of its 10th meeting, which was held December 12–13, 1998. As usual, we invited ten speakers from Japan and two guest speakers from abroad to the symposium, together with several leading Japanese hepatologists. Generally, there is no doubt that our technology for diagnosis and treatment of HCC is the best in the world. However, it is very important for us to exchange information with specialists in other parts of the world. Consequently, lectures on percutaneous ablation of HCC by Professor Tito Livraghi from Italy and on early detection of HCC by Professor Kwang-Hyub Han from Korea were very valuable in summarizing recent progress in HCC treatment. We can say that this proceedings, with its wealth of information on the treatment of HCC, is an important resource for physicians and hepatologists who are working in this specific field.

Finally, we thank the Otsuka Pharmaceutical Co., Ltd., for their continuing, helpful support.

ORGANIZING COMMITTEE OF THE YAMAGUCHI SYMPOSIUM
ON LIVER DISEASE
> Kiwamu Okita, M.D., Yamaguchi University, Ube
> Kenichi Kobayashi, M.D., Kanazawa University, Kanazawa
> Masamichi Kojiro, M.D., Kurume University, Kurume
> Masao Omata, M.D., University of Tokyo, Tokyo

Table of Contents

List of Participants

Fukumoto, Yohei   Department of General Internal Medicine
Yamaguchi University School of Medicine
Yamaguchi, Japan

Han, Kwang-Hyub   Department of Internal Medicine
Yonsei University
Seoul, Korea

Hayashi, Norio   Department of Molecular Therapeutics
Osaka University Faculty of Medicine
Osaka, Japan

Ichida, Fumihiro   Professor Emeritus
Niigata University School of Medicine
Niigata, Japan

Ichida, Takafumi   Third Department of Internal Medicine
Niigata University School of Medicine
Niigata, Japan

Kobayashi, Kenichi   First Department of Internal Medicine
Kanazawa University School of Medicine
Ishikawa, Japan

Kojiro, Masamichi   First Department of Pathology
Kurume University School of Medicine
Fukuoka, Japan

Kurokawa, Fumie   First Department of Internal Medicine
Yamaguchi University School of Medicine
Yamaguchi, Japan

Livraghi, Tito   Department of Radiology
Ospedale Civile Vimercate
Milano, Italy

Moriwaki, Hisataka   First Department of Internal Medicine
Gifu University School of Medicine
Gifu, Japan

Nakamura, Kenji	Department of Radiology Osaka City University Medical School Osaka, Japan
Nakanishi, Toshio	First Department of Internal Medicine Hiroshima University School of Medicine Hiroshima, Japan
Oka, Masaaki	Second Department of Surgery Yamaguchi University School of Medicine Yamaguchi, Japan
Okita, Kiwamu	First Department of Internal Medicine Yamaguchi University School of Medicine Yamaguchi, Japan
Omata, Masao	Department of Gastroenterology University of Tokyo Faculty of Medicine Tokyo, Japan
Sakaida, Isao	First Department of Internal Medicine Yamaguchi University School of Medicine Yamaguchi, Japan
Seki, Toshihito	Third Department of Internal Medicine Kansai Medical University Osaka, Japan
Shiina, Syuuichiro	Department of Gastroenterology University of Tokyo Faculty of Medicine Tokyo, Japan
Shirota, Yukihiro	First Department of Internal Medicine Kanazawa University School of Medicine Ishikawa, Japan
Tanaka, Masatoshi	Second Department of Internal Medicine Kurume University School of Medicine Fukuoka, Japan
Tanikawa, Kyuichi	Professor Emeritus Kurume University School of Medicine Fukuoka, Japan
Tatsumi, Tomohide	First Department of Internal Medicine Osaka University Faculty of Medicine Osaka, Japan

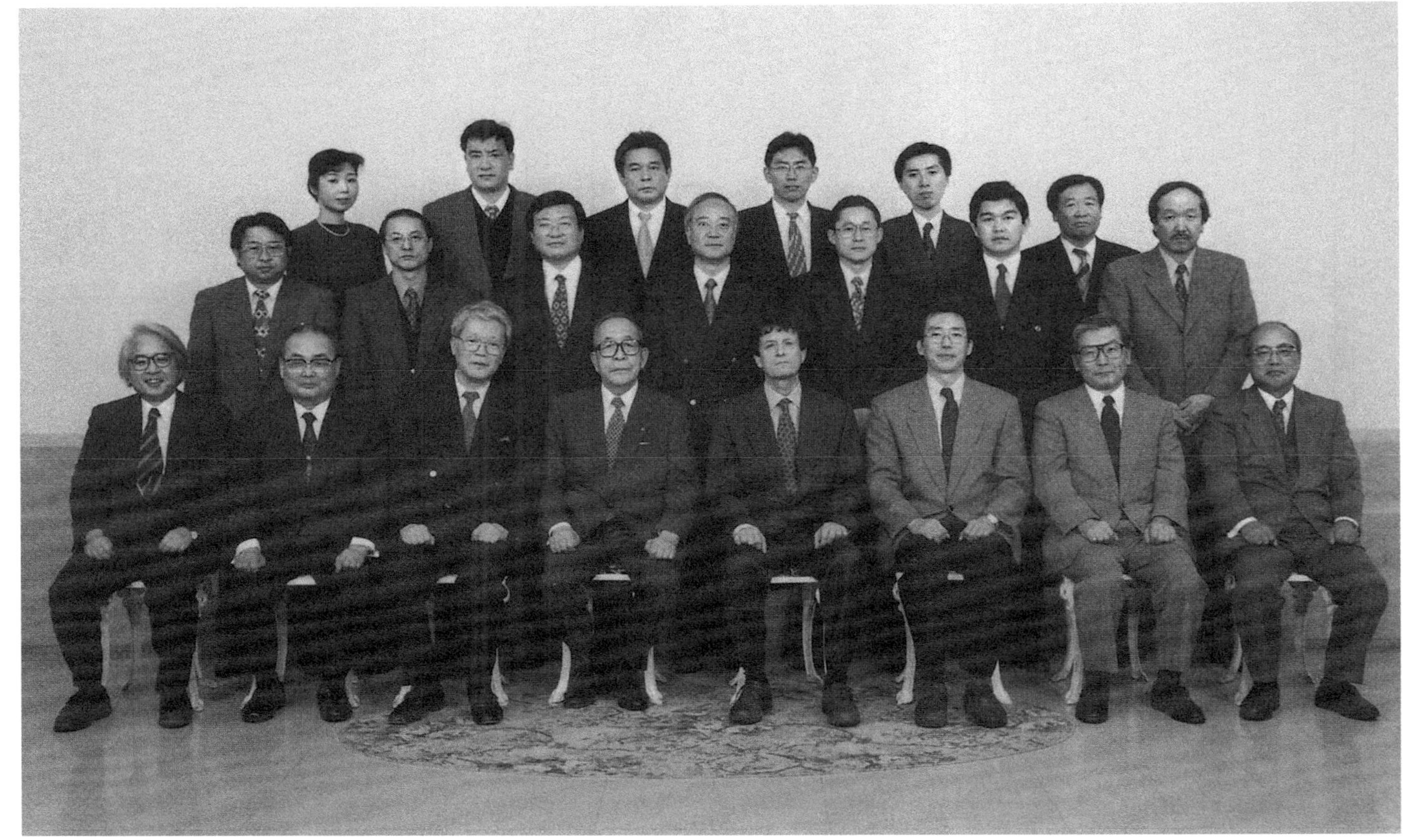

The Efficacy of the Ultrasonographic Screening Test for Early Detection of Hepatocellular Carcinoma and Risk Factors of HCC in Korea

Kwang-Hyub Han[1], Jeong Il Jeong[1], Sang Hoon Ahn[1], Dong Kee Kim[2], Chae Yoon Chon[1], and Young Myoung Moon[1]

Summary. To evaluate the effectiveness of screening for early detection of hepatocellular carcinoma (HCC) in Korea, the data of 12 899 patients who had ultrasonography (US) for reasons of chronic liver diseases were collected into a database program from 1990 to 1998. The risk factors of HCC were also studied. A total of 4 025 patients were enrolled who had repeated US. The male-to-female ratio was 2:1 and the age distribution was mostly between the fifth and seventh decades; 188 patients were diagnosed with HCC during follow-up (mean, 27 months), and the annual detection rate was 2.0%. The detection rate of small HCC ($\leq$3 cm in diameter) was 67.6%. The tumor size detected by screening within a 6-month interval was significantly smaller than at a longer interval (2.9 cm vs. 3.6 cm; $P < .01$). The smaller the tumor was at detection, the longer the survival time. Only 28.2% of HCC patients had an elevated serum alpha-fetoprotein (aFP) level above 400 ng/ml. The risk of HCC development during follow-up was higher among patients with liver cirrhosis (10.7%) than chronic hepatitis (4.0%) and higher for hepatitis C (8.8%) than hepatitis B (4.7%) and non-B, non-C hepatitis (non-BC, 3.7%). No cases of HCC developed at less than 30 years old, and there were none at less than 40 years among hepatitis C and non-BC. In conclusion, US screening within a 6-month interval is beneficial to high-risk patients over 40 years old through the early detection of HCC and prolonged survival. According to the risk factors, the necessity for a screening test and the proper interval should be reconsidered.

Key words. Ultrasonography, Screening test, Early diagnosis, Hepatocellular carcinoma, Risk factors

Introduction

As the prognosis of hepatocellular carcinoma (HCC) is extremely poor and an effective treatment for patients with advanced HCC has not yet been established, the early detection of HCC is important for effective treatment. Chronic hepatitis B and C as well as cirrhosis, irrespective of etiology, are recognized as the major

Departments of [1] Internal Medicine and [2] Biostatistics, Yonsei University Medical College, C.P.O. Box 8044, Seoul, Korea

factors increasing the risk of HCC [1–5]. Thus, screening has been extended to include patients with chronic hepatitis B or C as well as those with overt cirrhosis [5–8].

Although an HCC screening test has become an accepted procedure among high-risk populations, there are still some arguments about the effectiveness of screening because there has been no randomized controlled study showing a decrease in disease mortality [8–10]. In addition, the usefulness, frequency, and cost-effectiveness of screening for HCC may differ in different areas, which may reveal a different prevalence of hepatitis B or C.

HCC is the second most common malignancy and the second leading cause of death from cancer in Korea, where hepatitis B infection is highly endemic. The aim of this study was to evaluate the usefulness of a screening system in a clinic-based program for early diagnosis of HCC and to assess the risk factors of HCC development among Korean patients with chronic liver diseases.

Patients and Methods

Between January 1990 and January 1998, all the data of patients who had undergone ultrasonography (US) for reasons of screening for HCC or chronic liver diseases in our division of gastroenterology at Severance Hospital were collected into a special database program that we had designed. A total of 12 899 patients had 25 024 examinations during a period of 8 years and 1 month. We excluded patients with a history of liver cancer or other serious diseases that might affect survival. In addition, patients in whom focal hepatic lesion in the liver was the reason for the request for US and who were detected at initial examination or detected within 3 months after being enrolled were also excluded. All patients were periodically followed up by examinations at the outpatient clinic for liver disease at Severance Hospital. A total of 4 025 patients among those enrolled in this study had repeated US periodically for at least 1 more year.

To assess the risk factors of HCC development, the detailed data of clinical parameters in 1 467 patients among these were also collected by interview with a questionnaire and retrospective analysis of medical records. We also entered all detailed data into the database program. The male-to-female ratio was 2:1 and the age distribution was mostly between the fifth and seventh decades (Fig. 1). The clinical background of the patients was as follows: 76.8% of subjects were hepatitis B surface antigen (HBsAg) positive, 15.3% were anti-hepatitis C virus (anti-HCV) positive, 0.3% were positive for both, and 8.2% negative for both.

All patients were prospectively monitored by measurement of serum alpha-fetoprotein (aFP) and US at a 3- to 12-month interval according to the status of underlying liver disease. The mean follow-up duration was 27 ± 23 months, which was calculated by the US interval between the initial and final examination. The duration of HCC development was measured by the time interval between the date of initial US examination and diagnosis of HCC. When US showed a new focal lesion or serum aFP had increased, additional investigations were performed, such as a repeated test 1 month later, contrast computed tomography, or magnetic resonance imaging. HCC

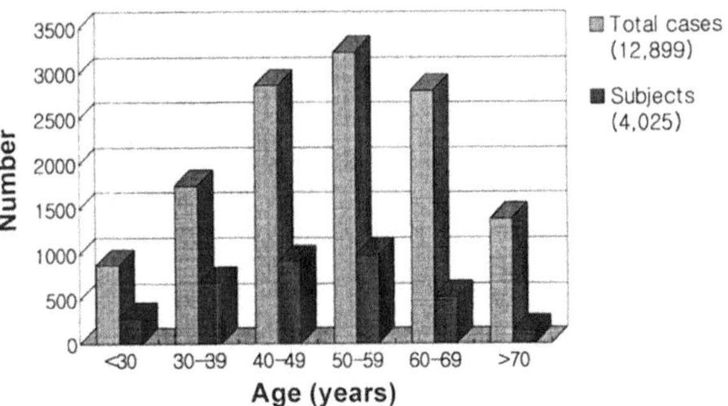

Fig. 1. Age distribution of study subjects who had repeated ultrasonography (US) periodically for at least 1 more year and total cases who had US for reasons of liver disease during the study period

was diagnosed by histological conformation or typical features on imaging diagnosis plus elevated serum aFP level ($\geq$400 ng/ml).

Serum aFP level was measured by a commercial enzyme-linked immunosorbent assay kit (Abbott, North Chicago, IL, USA). US was performed by internal physicians with high-resolution real-time US.

The data were analyzed statistically using the χ^2-test, logistic regression, or Kaplan–Meier method. All these statistical analyses were done by computer with the SAS program and SPSS for Windows (7.5.1) (Kaplan–Meier method and Cox regression hazard model).

Results

HCC was found in 182 patients by screening during follow-up (mean, 27 months), and the annual detection rate was 2.0%. At enrollment, the liver status of 140 patients (76.9%) of these was cirrhosis and 42 patients (23.1%) had chronic hepatitis. However, most patients (96.2%) progressed to liver cirrhosis at the time of detection of HCC (Table 1). Of 179 HCC patients, 128 (71.5%) were associated with hepatitis B, 35 patients (19.5%) were associated with hepatitis C, and 14 patients (7.8%) were unrelated to either hepatitis B or C (Table 2).

The mean diameter of tumor size at diagnosis was 3.3 $\pm$ 1.9 cm, and the detection rate of small HCC ($\leq$3 cm) was 67.6%; 16 of 148 patients (10.8%) had a tumor larger than 5 cm at diagnosis (Table 3). The mean diameter of the detected tumor by screening test within a 6-month interval was significantly smaller than at a longer interval (2.9 cm vs. 3.6 cm; $P < .01$). However, there was no size difference of tumor between a 3-month interval and a 3- to 6-month interval (Table 4). Median survival was 29 months (Table 5) and the smaller the tumor size was at detection, the longer was the survival time. Of 177 HCC patients, 50 (28.2%) had an elevated serum aFP level above 400 ng/ml at detection (Table 6). However, 71 patients (40.1%) had serum aFP levels below 20 ng/ml at diagnosis.

The incidence of HCC development was higher in patients with liver cirrhosis (10.7%) than in those with chronic hepatitis (4.0%) and in HBsAg carriers (1.3%). No patients with fatty liver developed HCC. The incidence of HCC development was

Table 1. Comparison of liver status at initial screening and at detection of hepatocellular carcinoma (HCC)

Liver status	No. of patients (%)	
	At initial screening	At detection of HCC
CH	42 (23.1)	7 (3.8)
LC	140 (76.9)	175 (96.2)
Child A	76 (41.8)	86 (47.3)
Child B	35 (19.2)	41 (22.5)
Child C	29 (15.9)	48 (26.4)

CH, chronic hepatitis; LC, liver cirrhosis.

Table 2. Underlying liver diseases at initial ultrasonography (US) of patients who developed HCC

Liver status	No. (%)				
	HBV(+)	HCV(+)	BC	Non-BC	Total
CH	30 (16.8)	9 (5.0)	1 (0.6)	2 (1.1)	42 (23.5)
LC	98 (54.7)	26 (14.5)	1 (0.6)	12 (6.7)	137 (76.5)
Total	128 (71.5)	35 (19.5)	2 (1.2)	14 (7.8)	179 (100.0)

CH, chronic hepatitis; LC, liver cirrhosis; BC, HBV(+) and HCV(+).

Table 3. Tumor size at diagnosis

Diameter (cm)	No. of patients (%)
≤2	60 (40.5)
>2–3	40 (27.1)
>3–5	32 (21.6)
>5	16 (10.8)
Total	148 (100.0)

Table 4. Tumor size according to US interval

US interval (months)	No. of patients (%)	Tumor size (cm)
≤6	83 (47.2)	2.9 ± 1.5*
≤3	18 (10.3)	3.6 ± 2.0
4–6	65 (36.9)	2.7 ± 1.3
>6	93 (52.8)	3.6 ± 2.2
7–12	65 (36.9)	3.2 ± 2.3
>12	28 (15.9)	4.6 ± 1.9
Total	176 (100.0)	3.3 ± 1.9

*, $P < .01$ vs. >6-month group.

Table 5. Median survival according to tumor size

Diameter	No. of patients (%)	Median survival (months)*
≤2 cm	60 (40.5)	40
>2–3 cm	40 (27.1)	33
>3–5 cm	32 (21.6)	18
>5 cm	16 (10.8)	8
Total	148 (100.0)	29

*, $P < .001$.

Table 6. Serum alpha-fetoprotein (aFP) level at detection of HCC

aFP level (ng/ml)	No. of patients (%)
≤20	71 (40.1)
21–400	56 (31.6)
>400	50 (28.2)

higher in the hepatitis C-related group (8.8%) than the hepatitis B- (4.7%) and non-B, non-C hepatitis (non-BC) -related group (3.7%). However, there was no significant difference between hepatitis C and B patients who were older than 40 years. No cases HCC developed below the age of 30 years, and there were none below 40 years among hepatitis C- and non-BC-related groups.

Discussion

In Korea, HCC is the second most common malignancy (11.7% of registered cancer patients; 1996 Korean National Cancer Registry). Annual deaths from HCC were 21.4 per 100 000 Korean population, which was the second leading cause of deaths from cancer in Korea (1996 report of Korean National Statistical Office). As Korea is a highly endemic area of hepatitis B infection, about 70% of Korean patients with HCC were hepatitis B related.

The usefulness, frequency, and cost-effectiveness of screening for HCC may differ in different geographic areas or among different underlying liver disease populations because there may be differences in the incidence and growth characteristics [8,9]. Although US screening for HCC is still controversial for improving survival of HCC, it is a generally accepted strategy in East Asian countries.

Cirrhosis is recognized as the major risk factor for HCC, and the annual risk of developing HCC is between 1% and 6% [2,4,11–15]. In our study, the annual risk of HCC in cirrhosis was 3.5%. Reported screening studies have mostly focused on cirrhotic patients as the target population. However, 20% to 56% of patients presenting with HCC have previously undiagnosed cirrhosis [16,17]. Thus, screening has been extended to include patients with chronic viral hepatitis as well as those with overt cirrhosis. The overall reported annual detection rate of HCC in surveillance studies including chronic hepatitis varied from 0.8% to 4.1% [3,9,18–22]. In our study, the annual detection rate in chronic hepatitis was 1.19%.

If the sample size of the target population or the number of HCC cases that were detected is not large enough, it is difficult to evaluate the effectiveness of screening in a high-risk population with different status and etiology of liver diseases. Therefore, a large target population and a sufficient number of HCC detected by screening can avoid sampling bias. In our study, the study subjects were enrolled from 12 899 patients who had US for HCC screening or various chronic liver diseases in our division. We enrolled 4 025 patients who had repeated US periodically for a period of at least 1 year longer by using a database program. Our study included a variety of liver diseases such as hepatitis B or C carriers, chronic hepatitis, fatty liver, and liver cirrhosis related to hepatitis B, C, or non-BC. We found 182 patients with HCC during a mean 27-month follow-up, and the annual detection rate was 2.0%.

As the sample size was enough large to allow estimation, we tried to evaluate the efficacy of screening for HCC in various liver disease groups. Because our study was a clinic-based screening, the incidence of HCC development was higher than that reported by Sherman et al. [8], who detected 14 tumors among 1 069 hepatitis B virus (HBV) carriers by US screening in a North American urban population. In our study, 76.9% of patients with HCC had liver cirrhosis and 23.1% had chronic hepatitis at the time they were enrolled in the study. Furthermore, most of these cases progressed to liver cirrhosis during follow-up and before development of HCC. Although the incidence of HCC development was higher in liver cirrhosis (10.7%) than chronic hepatitis (4.0%) cases, chronic hepatitis B or C might progress to cirrhosis and develop HCC during long-term follow-up. Thus, surveillance is needed to include patients with chronic viral hepatitis over the age of 40 in Korea.

Reported screening intervals vary from 3 to 12 months. A 6-month interval is generally accepted as a rational choice [23,24]. However, some others prefer shorter intervals in a high-risk population such as cirrhotic patients to allow detection an earlier stage [25]. In our study, the mean diameter of tumor size at diagnosis was 3.3 ± 1.9 cm and the detection rate of small HCC (<3 cm) was 67.6%, which was comparable with other studies. Especially, the mean diameter of the detected tumor size by screening test within a 6-month interval was significantly smaller than at a longer interval (2.9 cm vs. 3.6 cm; $P < .01$). However, there was no size difference between a 3-month interval and within a 3- to 6-month interval (see Table 4), which means a 6-month-interval US screening is adequate to diagnose HCC in an early stage. Although the shorter screening interval offers a better chance to detect HCC earlier, cost-effectiveness can decrease.

There is still an unresolved question as to whether an apparent improvement in survival by screening is the result of early detection or lead-time bias [9]. In our study, overall median survival of the screened group was 29 months, which was longer than the 7 months survival of 578 nonscreened HCC patients in our institute (data not shown). Survival time correlated well with tumor size at detection. Furthermore, survival time can be remarkably improved when the detected tumor size is equal or smaller than 2 cm (see Table 5). Although the resection rate was relatively low in our study, most tumors, especially those less than 3 cm, were amenable to nonsurgical curative or effective therapy.

Only 50 of 177 HCC patients (28.2%) had an elevated serum aFP level, that is, above 400 ng/ml at detection. In addition, the serum aFP level in 40.1% of patients was below 20 ng/ml at diagnosis. Therefore, serum aFP alone is not adequate for use as a screening program in Korea.

The incidence of HCC development was higher in liver cirrhosis (10.7%) than in chronic hepatitis (4.0%). None of the patients with fatty liver developed HCC. The incidence of HCC development was higher in the hepatitis C-related group (8.8%) than the hepatitis B- (4.7%) and non-BC-related groups (3.7%). However, the incidence was not significantly different between hepatitis C and B in the group over 40 years of age.

No study has yet directly addressed the question of whether surveillance for HCC should be restricted to individuals over a certain age limit. In our study, there were no cases of HCC developed below 30 years old and there were none below 40 years among hepatitis C and non-BC. As the risk of HCC is negligible before the age of 30 in hepatitis B and the age of 40 in hepatitis C, the screening would be better restricted to patients over 40 years.

In conclusion, the US screening test within a 6-month interval is beneficial to high-risk patients more than 40 years old through early detection of HCC and prolonged survival. According to risk factors, the necessity for a screening test and proper interval should be reconsidered.

We would suggest a more cost-effective screening test through the evaluation of the relative risk factors of HCC development among the risk group for HCC. Our database program will be useful to manage the data of patients taking the screening test.

Acknowledgments. This study was supported by a grant of the 1997–1998 Korean National Cancer Control Program, Ministry of Health & Welfare, R.O.K.

References

1. Beasley RP, Hwang LU, Lin CC, Chien CS (1981) Hepatocellular carcinoma and hepatitis B virus: a prospective study of 22707 men in Taiwan. Lancet 2:1129–1133
2. Kato Y, Nakata K, Omagari K, Furukawa R, Kusumoto Y, Mori I, Tajima H, Tanioka H, Yano M, Nagtak S (1994) Risk of hepatocellular carcinoma in patients with cirrhosis in Japan. Cancer (Phila) 74:2234–2238
3. Takano S, Yokosuka O, Imazeki F, Tagawa M, Omata M (1995) Incidence of hepatocellular carcinoma in chronic hepatitis B and C: a prospective study of 251 patients. Hepatology 21:650–655
4. Ikeda K, Saitoh S, Koida I, Arase Y, Tsubota A, Chayama K, Kumada H, Kawanishi M (1993) A multivariate analysis of risk factors for hepatocellular carcinoma: a prospective observation of 795 patients with viral and alcoholic cirrhosis. Hepatology 18: 47–53

5. Bruix J, Barrera JM, Calvert X, Ercilla G, Costa J, Sanchez-Tapias JM, Ventura M, Vall M, Bruguera M, Bru C (1989) Prevalence of antibodies to hepatitis C virus in Spanish patients with hepatocellular carcinoma and hepatitis cirrhosis. Lancet 2:1004–1005
6. Villenuve J-P, Desrochers M, Infante-Rivard C, Willems B, Raymond G, Bourcier M, Cote J, Richer G (1994) A long-term follow-up study of asymptomatic hepatitis B surface antigen-positive carriers in Montreal. Gastroenterology 108:1000–1005
7. McMahon BJ, Alberts SR, Wainwright RB, Bulkow L, Lanier AP (1990) Hepatitis B-related sequelae. Prospective study of 1 400 hepatitis B surface antigen-positive Alaska native carriers. Arch Intern Med 150:1051–1054
8. Sherman M, Peltekian KM, Lee C (1995) Screening for hepatocellular carcinoma in chronic carriers of hepatitis B virus: incidence and prevalence of hepatocellular carcinoma in a North American urban population. Hepatology 22:432–438
9. Collier J, Sherman M (1998) Screening for hepatocellular carcinoma. Hepatology 27:273–277
10. Di Bisceglie AM, Carithers RL, Gores GJ (1998) Hepatocellular carcinoma. Hepatology 28:1161–1165
11. Colombo M, De Franchis R, Del Ninno E, Sangiovanni A, De Fazio C, Tommasini M, Donato MF, Piva A, Di Carlo V, Dioguardi N (1991) Hepatocellular carcinoma in Italian patients with cirrhosis. Lancet 325:675–680
12. Cottone M, Turri M, Caltagirone M, Prisi P, Orlando A, Fiorentino G, Virdone R, Fusco G, Grasso R, Simonetti RG (1994) Screening for hepatocellular carcinoma in patients with Child's A cirrhosis: an 8-year prospective study by ultrasound and alpha-fetoprotein. J Hepatol (Amst) 21:1029–1034
13. Oka H, Tamori A, Juroki T, Kobayashi K, Yamamoto S (1994) Prospective study of alpha-fetoprotein in cirrhotic patients monitored for development of hepatocellular carcinoma. Hepatology 19:61–66
14. Zaman SN, Melia WM, Johnson RD, Portmann BC, Johnson PJ, Williams R (1985) Risk factors in development of hepatocellular carcinoma in cirrhosis: prospective study of 613 patients. Lancet 1:1357–1360
15. Pateron D, Ganne N, Trinchet JC, Aurousseau MH, Mal F, Meicler C, Coderc E, Reboullet P, Beaugrand M (1994) Prospective study of screening for hepatocellular carcinoma in Caucasian patients with cirrhosis. J Hepatol 20:65–71
16. The Liver Cancer Study Group of Japan (1990) Primary liver cancer in Japan. Clinicopathologic features and results of surgical treatment. Ann Surg 211:277–287
17. Zaman SN, Johnson PJ, Williams R (1990) Silent cirrhosis in patients with hepatocellular carcinoma. Implications for screening in high-incidence and low-incidence areas. Cancer (Phila) 65:1607–1610
18. Liaw Y-F, Tai D-I, Chu C-M, Lin D-Y, Sheen I-S, Chen T-J, Pao CC (1986) Early detection of hepatocellular carcinoma in patients with chronic type B hepatitis. Gastroenterology 90:263–266
19. Chiba T, Matsuzaki Y, Abei M, Shoda J, Tanaka N, Osuga T, Aikawa T (1996) The role of previous hepatits B virus infection and heavy smoking in hepatitis C virus-related hepatocellular carcinoma. Am J Gastroenterol 91:1195–1211
20. Tanaka S, Kitamura T, Nakanishi K, Okuda S, Yamazaki H, Hiyama T, Fujimoto I (1990) Effectiveness of periodic checkup by ultrasonography for the early diagnosis of hepatocellular carcinoma. Cancer (Phila) 66:2110–2214
21. Curley SA, Izzo F, Gallipoli A, de Bellis M, Cremona F, Parisi V (1995) Identification and screening of 416 patients with chronic hepatitis at high risk to develop hepatocellular carcinoma. Ann Surg 222:375–383
22. Tsukuma H, Hiyama T, Tanaka S, Nakao M, Yabuuchi T, Kitamura T, Nakanishi K, Fujimoto I, Inoue A, Yamazaki H, Kawashima T (1993) Risk factors for hepatocellular carcinoma among patients with chronic liver disease. N Engl J Med 328:1797–1801

23. Chen DS, Sung JL, Sheu JC, Lau MY, How SW, Hsu HC, Lee CS, Wei TC (1984) Serum alpha fetoprotein in the early stage of human hepatocellular carcinoma. Gastroenterology 86:1404–1409
24. Sheu JC, Sung JL, Chen DS, Yang PM, Lau MY, Lee CS, Hsu HC, Chung CN, Yang PC, Wang TH, Lin JT, Lee CZ (1984) Growth rates of asymptomatic hepatocellular carcinoma and its clinical implication. Gastroenterology 86:1404–1409

Percutaneous Ethanol Injection Therapy, Percutaneous Infarction Therapy, and Percutaneous Microwave Coagulation Therapy for Hepatocellular Carcinoma

SHUICHIRO SHIINA, TAKUMA TERATANI, MASATOSHI IMAMURA, SHUNTARO OBI, SHINPEI SATO, YUKIHIRO KOIKE, TAKAYUKI DAN, MASATOSHI AKAMATSU, TOMONORI FUJISHIMA, NAOYA KATO, YASUO IMAI, KEISUKE HAMAMURA, YASUSHI SHIRATORI, and MASAO OMATA

Summary. Nonsurgical treatments play important roles in the treatment of hepatocellular carcinoma. At our institute, more than 90% of new patients with hepatocellular carcinoma have been treated by percutaneous ethanol injection therapy (PEIT) or other percutaneous tumor ablations. Here we describe our experience in those procedures. Between 1985 and 1997, we performed PEIT on 653 patients, and the 1-, 3-, 5-, and 10-year survival rates were 89%, 63%, 38%, and 18%. In 349 patients who had three or fewer lesions and all of whose lesions were 3 cm or less in diameter, the survival rates were 93%, 74%, 47%, and 26% at 1, 3, 5, and 10 years. In percutaneous infarction therapy (PIT), ethanol is injected into the feeding artery, as detected by color Doppler ultrasonography, to cut off the blood flow to the tumor. Successful PIT induces infarction of an area in which the lesion is located. We performed PIT on 18 patients and achieved infarction in 17 of them. PIT is especially useful for a large lesion located in a peripheral portion of the liver. Percutaneous microwave coagulation therapy (PMCT) is a therapy in which heat produced by microwave energy emitted from the inserted electrode destroys the cancer tissue. Using an introducing needle with a scale, a stopper for the electrode, and a guide needle, we performed PMCT on 108 patients. CT scan following the therapy demonstrated complete necrosis of the lesion in 94 cases. Effective mass reduction was accomplished in the remaining 14 cases in which PMCT was used only palliatively. PMCT can surely destroy a certain amount of tissue, although its necrotic area is smaller than that of PEIT. Percutaneous tumor ablation techniques seem useful for hepatocellular carcinoma treatment.

Key words. Percutaneous ethanol injection therapy, Percutaneous infarction therapy, Percutaneous microwave coagulation therapy, Hepatocellular carcinoma

Department of Gastroenterology, University of Tokyo, Hongo 7-3-1, Bunkyo-ku, Tokyo 113-0033, Japan

Introduction

Hepatocellular carcinoma is different from other solid tumors because surgery plays a limited role. The resectability rate of this cancer is low because of multiple lesions or underlying cirrhosis [1]. Still worse, the cancer frequently recurs even after curative surgical resection [2,3]. Thus, nonsurgical therapies play important roles in the treatment of hepatocellular carcinoma.

At our institute, more than 90% of new patients with hepatocellular carcinoma have been treated by percutaneous ethanol injection therapy (PEIT) or other percutaneous tumor ablations. We describe here our experience in percutaneous ethanol injection therapy, percutaneous infarction therapy (PIT), and percutaneous microwave coagulation therapy (PMCT) for hepatocellular carcinoma.

Percutaneous Ethanol Injection Therapy (PEIT)

Introduction of PEIT brought about a drastic change in the treatment of hepatocellular carcinoma [4]. It has enabled us to treat hepatocellular carcinoma effectively by nonsurgical measures [5-12]. Histopathologic examinations after the therapy have revealed that PEIT can destroy the tumor completely in most cases [8]. PEIT has achieved high long-term survival rates [9-11]. For small hepatocellular carcinoma, PEIT has been generally accepted as an alternative to surgery in Japan [12].

Between 1985 and 1997, 721 new patients with hepatocellular carcinoma were hospitalized at our institute, and among these, 653 patients (91%) were treated by PEIT.

Indications of PEIT are as follows:

1. Unresectable lesions or preference for nonsurgical therapies
2. Absence of apparent vascular or biliary invasion
3. Three or fewer hypervascular lesions or hypovascular lesions
4. Absence of uncontrollable ascites
5. Absence of marked bleeding tendency (prothrombin times should be 35% or more, and platelet count should be 40 000/mm^3 or more).
6. Serum bilirubin level of less than 4.0 mg/dl,
7. Receipt of informed consent.

Patient age ranged from 35 to 87 years (mean 62 years), and 83% had cirrhosis. A single lesion was present in 321 cases, two lesions in 139 cases, three lesions in 66 cases, and four or more lesions in 127 cases. Lesion size was 1.0 cm or less in 22 cases, 1.1–2.0 cm in 180 cases, 2.1–3.0 cm in 209 cases, 3.1–5.0 cm in 184 cases, and 5.1 cm or more in 58 cases. PEIT alone was performed in 513 cases (79%) and combined with transcatheter arterial embolization in 140 cases.

We used the multiple-needle insertion technique to perform PEIT [13]. By inserting multiple needles and changing the depth of the tip of the needles, we can inject ethanol into several portions in one treatment session. In some cases, we also used PEIT with CT assistance. In this method, we first insert needles under ultrasound guidance, and then we use CT to confirm that the tip of the needle is at the intended site. By using the multiple-needle insertion technique and the CT assistance method, we can use PEIT against lesions of more than 5 cm diameter, and thus we can treat more than 90% of patients with hepatocellular carcinoma by PEIT.

PEIT was performed twice a week, until it was considered that ethanol had been injected throughout the lesion. Then, CT was performed to determine whether there was any viable cancer tissue or not. If viable cancer tissue was detected, PEIT was repeated until CT confirmed that the entire tumor had become necrotic.

With regard to the long-term efficacy, the survival rates of all 653 patients treated by PEIT were 89% at 1 year, 63% at 3 years, 38% at 5 years, and 18% at 10 years (Fig. 1). In 349 patients who had three or fewer lesions and all of whose lesions were 3 cm or less in diameter, the survival rates were 93% at 1 year, 74% at 3 years, 47% at 5 years, and 26% at 10 years. Furthermore, in 523 patients in which all lesions detected by imaging modalities were treated by PEIT as potentially curative treatment, the survival rates were 93% at 1 year, 70% at 3 years, 46% at 5 years, and 25% at 10 years (Fig. 2). In the remaining 130 patients, which we call the noncurable group, only the main

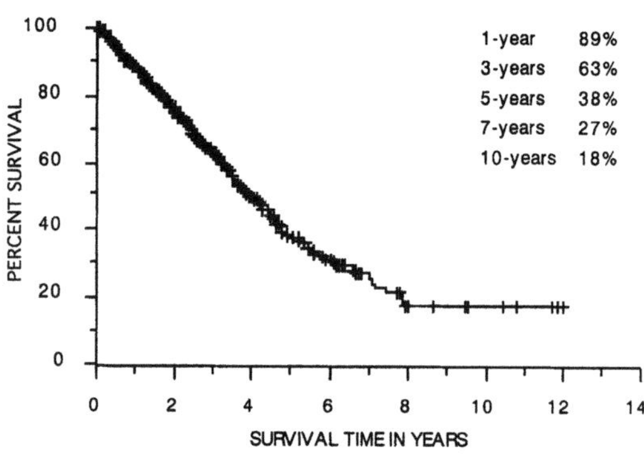

Fig. 1. Survival rates of all 653 patients treated by percutaneous ethanol injection therapy

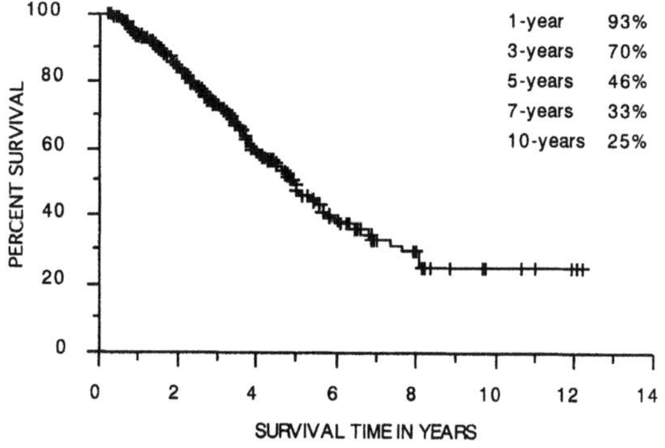

Fig. 2. Survival rates of 523 patients in which all lesions detected by imaging modalities were treated by percutaneous ethanol injection therapy as curative treatment

lesions were treated by PEIT, some being left untreated by PEIT because of the large number of lesions.

Complications encountered were peritoneal bleeding in 8 cases, seeding of the cancer cells in 8 cases, hemobilia in 6 cases, massive hepatic infarction in 3 cases, and others. There was one operational mortality.

In PEIT, injected ethanol is distributed in a limited area and the distribution may not be homogeneous even within this area because of the capsule and septa of the lesion. Furthermore, if an excessive amount of ethanol flows out of the lesion, it may damage noncancerous liver tissue.

On the other hand, PEIT can destroy a relatively large area inside the capsule in one ablation. Thus, PEIT can be used for lesions over 3 cm in diameter. Furthermore, if necessary, PEIT can be performed for lesions which can be approached only by penetrating vessels, because the needles used in PEIT are relatively small (21 or 22 gauge). Moreover, PEIT can also be performed for lesions which move markedly during respiration because the needle need only be kept in one place for a few seconds. PEIT can also be performed for lesions in delicate places, because the tip of the needle is clearly seen by ultrasound. In conclusion, PEIT has very wide indications in the treatment of hepatocellular carcinoma.

Percutaneous Infarction Therapy (PIT)

PIT is a therapy using color Doppler ultrasonography [14]. Recent advances in color Doppler ultrasonography have made it possible to detect the arteries feeding hepatocellular carcinoma. By injecting ethanol into the feeding artery and cutting off the blood flow, infarction can be induced in the area in which the lesion is located. PIT is indicated for patients in which the arterial signal is still detected in the feeding artery despite several applications of PEIT.

We performed PIT in 18 patients with lesions ranging from 2.1 cm to 8.4 cm in diameter. PIT was performed on the main lesion in all cases, and other lesions were treated by PEIT.

The procedure is as follows:

1. Detection of the feeding artery by color Doppler ultrasonography, and insertion of a 21-gauge needle.
2. Confirmation of the reflux of the arterial blood flow through the needle.
3. Slow injection of ethanol until the arterial signal disappears.
4. On recanalization of the feeding artery, the same procedure is repeated.
5. Execution of a CT scan to evaluate the distribution of necrosis after hepatic infarction is generated.

Infarction of the area in which the tumor was located was induced in 17 of the 18 cases. The number of treatment sessions ranged from 1 to 8. Complications encountered were bronchobiliary fistula and cholangitis. In conclusion, PIT is especially useful for a large lesion located in a peripheral portion of the liver.

Percutaneous Microwave Coagulation Therapy (PMCT)

PMCT is a therapy in which heat produced by microwave energy emitted from the inserted electrode destroys the cancer tissue [15]. It can destroy a certain amount of tissue, although its necrotic area is smaller than that of PEIT.

Indications of PMCT are somewhat different from those of PEIT. Because a relatively large introducing needle is used in PMCT, prothrombin time should be 50% or more and the platelet count should be at least $50\,000/mm^3$. In addition, and serum bilirubin level should be less than 2.0 mg/dl. Indications of PMCT is limited for lesions located in portions of the liver where the electrode can be inserted and held safely.

PMCT was performed in 108 patients with hepatocellular carcinoma. PMCT was used for the initial lesion in 60 cases and for recurrent lesions in 48 cases. There was a single lesion in 66 cases, two lesions in 22 cases, three lesions in 11 cases, and four or more lesions in 9 cases. The size was 1.0 cm or less in 4 cases, 1.1–2.0 cm in 36 cases, 2.1–3.0 cm in 34 cases, 3.1–5.0 cm in 24 cases, and 5.1 cm or more in 10 cases. PMCT alone was performed in 68 cases and combined with PEIT or transcatheter arterial embolization in 40 cases.

Under US-guidance, introducing needles were first inserted and then the electrode was inserted through the needles. Radiation for dielectric heating was performed at 65–85 W for 60 s.

Enhanced CT scans were was done in all 108 cases to evaluate the therapeutic effect of PMCT. Complete necrosis of the lesion with some safety margin was achieved in 94 cases. Effective mass reduction was accomplished in the remaining 14 cases in which PMCT was used only palliatively. Long-term survival rates have not been analyzed because of the short observation period. Local recurrence of the treated lesions within 18 months was encountered in 4 cases.

No complications were encountered in 90 cases, massive pleural effusion in 7 cases, hemobilia in 3 cases, hemothorax in 2 cases, hemoperitoneum in 2 cases, and others. Complications frequently occurred in the middle of our study during which time we increased the number of ablations to completely destroy all lesions in one day. Recently, however, complications have been rare.

PMCT has a weak point in that its necrotic area is relatively small; the resulting size of necrosis is about 1.5 cm in diameter and 2.5 cm in length. Complete necrosis can be assured only in lesions up to 1 cm in diameter if ablation is done only in the center of the lesion. In large lesions, the electrode should be inserted into various portions in the lesion. However, once ablation has been carried out, the lesion becomes difficult to observe because of the gas bubbles generated, and the electrode cannot be inserted precisely for repeat therapy.

Our multiple-needle insertion technique has been successful in PEIT, precisely injecting ethanol into each portion of the lesion. We wanted to try a similar technique for PMCT. Thus we made an introducing needle with a scale, a stopper for the electrode, and a guide needle with a scale [16]. With these tools, the electrode can be inserted into each portion in the lesion systematically.

With PMCT it is easy to achieve complete necrosis with some safety margin in small or medium-size liver tumors because, unlike PEIT, heat effects are not limited by the capsule or septa. However, if PMCT is performed without care, viable cancer tissue may remain even inside the capsule. Lesions over 3 cm in diameter are difficult to treat by PMCT alone because one ablation by PMCT can produce only a small area of necrosis. Furthermore, lesions which can be approached only by penetrating vessels are excluded from PMCT because thick introducing needles (14 gauge) are necessary. Heat transmitted by introducing needles and the electrode often damages the puncture track and causes complications, such as pleural effusion. In conclusion, PMCT is useful in the treatment of hepatocellular carcinoma, although there are still various problems to be solved.

Conclusion

Various percutaneous tumor ablation techniques are available for hepatocellular carcinoma. The strong points and weak points of each therapy must be understood and the most appropriate therapy chosen for each patient. Percutaneous tumor ablation techniques play essential roles in the treatment of hepatocellular carcinoma.

References

1. Liver Cancer Study Group of Japan (1998) Survey and follow-up study of primary liver cancer in Japan: report 13 (in Japanese). Shinko-insatsu, Kyoto, pp 13–14
2. Nagasue N, Yukaya H, Ogawa Y, Sasaki Y, Chang YG, Niimi K (1986) Clinical experience with 118 hepatic resections for hepatocellular carcinoma. Surgery 99:694–701
3. Lin TY, Lee CS, Chen KM, Chen CC (1987) Role of surgery in the treatment of primary carcinoma of the liver: a 31-year experience. Br J Surg 74:839–842
4. Sugiura N, Takara K, Ohto M, Okuda K, Hirooka N (1983) Percutaneous intratumoral injection of ethanol under ultrasound imaging for treatment of small hepatocellular carcinoma (in Japanese). Acta Hepatol Jpn 24:920
5. Livraghi T, Festi D, Monti F, Salmi A, Vettori C (1986) US-guided percutaneous alcohol injection of small hepatic and abdominal tumors. Radiology 161:309–312
6. Shiina S, Yasuda H, Muto H, Tagawa K, Unuma T, Ibukuro K, Inoue Y, Takanashi R (1987) Percutaneous ethanol injection in the treatment of liver neoplasms. AJR 149: 949–952
7. Sheu JC, Sung JL, Huang GT, Chen DS, Yang PM, Lai MY, Wei TC, Su CT, Tsang YM, Lee CZ (1987) Intratumor injection of absolute ethanol under ultrasound guidance for the treatment of small hepatocellular carcinoma. Hepatogastroenterology 34:255–261
8. Shiina S, Tagawa K, Unuma T, Takanashi R, Yoshiura K, Komatsu Y, Hata Y, Niwa Y, Shiratori Y, Terano A, Sugimoto T (1991) Percutaneous ethanol injection therapy for hepatocellular carcinoma: a histopathologic study. Cancer 68:1524–1530
9. Ebara M, Ohto M, Sugiura N, Kita K, Yoshikawa M, Okuda K, Kondo F, Kondo Y (1990) Percutaneous ethanol injection for the treatment of small hepatocellular carcinoma: study of 95 patients. J Gastroenterol Hepatol 5:616–626
10. Shiina S, Tagawa K, Niwa Y, Unuma T, Komatsu Y, Yoshiura K, Hamada E, Takahashi M, Shiratori Y, Terano A, Omata M, Kawauchi N, Inoue H (1993) Percutaneous ethanol injection therapy for hepatocellular carcinoma: results in 146 patients. AJR 160:1023–1028

11. Livraghi T, Giorgio A, Marin G, Salmi A, de-Sio I, Bolondi L, Pompili M, Brunello F, Lazzaroni S, Torzilli G (1995) Hepatocellular carcinoma and cirrhosis in 746 patients: long-term results of percutaneous ethanol injection. Radiology 197:101–108
12. Shiina S, Imamura M, Omata M (1997) Percutaneous ethanol injection therapy (PEIT) for malignant liver neoplasms. Semin Intervent Radiol 14:295–303
13. Shiina S, Hata Y, Niwa Y (1991) Multiple-needle insertion method in percutaneous ethanol injection therapy for liver neoplasms. Gastroenterologia Jpn 26:47–50
14. Imamura M, Shiratori Y, Shiina S (1998) Percutaneous hepatic infarction therapy for hepatocellular caricnoma. AJR 171:1031–1035
15. Seki T, Wakabayashi M, Nakagawa T (1994) Ultrasonically guided percutaneous microwave coagulation therapy for small hepatocellular carcinoma. Cancer 74:817–825
16. Shiina S, Imamura M, Obi S (1997) Percutaneous microwave coagulation therapy for liver neoplasms (in Japanese). J Microware Surg 15:65–69

Percutaneous Microwave Coagulation Therapy for Hepatocellular Carcinoma

TOSHIHITO SEKI, TAIICHI NAKAGAWA, TORU TAMAI, MASATO IMAMURA, AKIRA NISHIMURA, NORIYO YAMASHIKI, MASAYUKI WAKABAYASHI, and KYOICHI INOUE

Summary. We introduce the microwave coagulation system and the technique of percutaneous microwave coagulation therapy (PMCT) and report the effect of PMCT for small hepatocellular carcinoma (HCC). We used PMCT as a new percutaneous local treatment for single HCC measuring 2 cm or less in diameter (small HCC). We performed PMCT on 59 patients with small HCC. The 5-year survival rate was 70% and the 5-year disease-free survival rate was 22%. Serious complications have not been experienced in this study. PMCT appears to be a safe and effective treatment for solitary small liver cancer.

Key words. Hepatocellular carcinoma, Microwave coagulation, Percutaneous local treatment

Introduction

As the initial treatment for small hepatocellular carcinoma (HCC), surgical resection, transcatheter arterial embolization (TAE) [1], and ultrasonography- (US) guided local treatment have been performed alone or in combination. Surgical resection is not a viable option for all patients because they may have poor liver function induced by liver cirrhosis. Furthermore, TAE is sometimes ineffective because of inadequate angioneogenesis in small HCC [2]. For these reasons, US-guided percutaneous local treatment has been adopted independently or in combination with TAE. We formulated US-guided percutaneous microwave coagulation therapy (PMCT) as a new method of percutaneous local treatment to induce complete tumor necrosis. In this chapter, we present our clinical data using PMCT alone for small HCCs.

Third Department of Internal Medicine, Kansai Medical University, 10-15 Fumizonocho, Moriguchi, Osaka 570-8507, Japan

Methods and Patients

Treatment Modalities

Microwave Electrode

The custom-made electrode used was 2.0 mm in diameter and 25 cm long. At the electrode terminus, 1 cm of the inner conductor is exposed and is insulated from the circular outer conductor by polytetrafluorethylene. The conductor is stainless steel.

Power Output Assessment of Microwave Delivery System

An in vitro evaluation of heat dissipation was performed by assessing temperature changes in eggwhite heated by the microwave electrode and microwave generator (Microtaze OT-110M; Nippon Shoji, Osaka, Japan). The extent of heating was measured using a thermographic camera (Infra-eye 180; Fujitsu, Tokyo, Japan). Eggwhite in a glass chamber was heated by microwaves. With irradiation at 80 W for 60 s, it was possible to raise the temperature to more than 64°C in an area 3.5–4.0 cm in maximal diameter and 2.5–3.0 cm in minimal diameter.

The coagulation of normal rabbit liver by microwaves was then tested. Five healthy, fasting adult white rabbits (mean weight, 2.5 kg) were used. They were immobilized in the supine position and placed under ketamine hydrochloride (1 mg/kg, i.m.) anesthesia. The right hepatic lobe was exposed via a median incision on the abdomen. The microwave electrode was inserted into the right lobe and the area was irradiated at 80 W for 60 s. The abdomen was then closed. The animals were killed 3 days later and the coagulated areas were observed. The coagulated area was elliptical, with maximal and minimal diameters (mean ± SD) of 3.1 ± 0.5 and 2.2 ± 0.4 cm, respectively.

With regard to the irradiation time, 60 s is optimal for obtaining the maximal coagulated area. Even if the microwave irradiation continues for more than 60 s, the coagulated area is much the same as that obtained with 60 s of irradiation.

Percutaneous Microwave Coagulation Therapy

PMCT (Fig. 1) was performed in accordance with the method previously employed [3]. After local anesthesia, a 13-gauge, 15-cm-long guide needle (Guiding Needle; Hakko, Tokyo, Japan) was inserted in the vicinity of the tumor with the aid of sonographic guidance [3.5-MHz microconvex probe (SSD-2000), Aloka, Tokyo, or 3.75-MHz microconvex probe (SSA-260A), Toshiba, Tokyo, Japan]. The inner needle of the guide was then removed, and the microwave electrode was inserted through the outer needle of the guide to place the electrode in the tumor area. The electrode was connected to a microwave generator via a flexible coaxial cable. The tumor area was then irradiated with microwaves at 80 W for 60 s. Following irradiation of the tumor area with microwaves, the electrode and the outer needle of the guide were removed. Microwave irradiation at 80 W was administered to the puncture track (from the treated area to the site near the liver surface) for about 10–20 s to prevent bleeding,

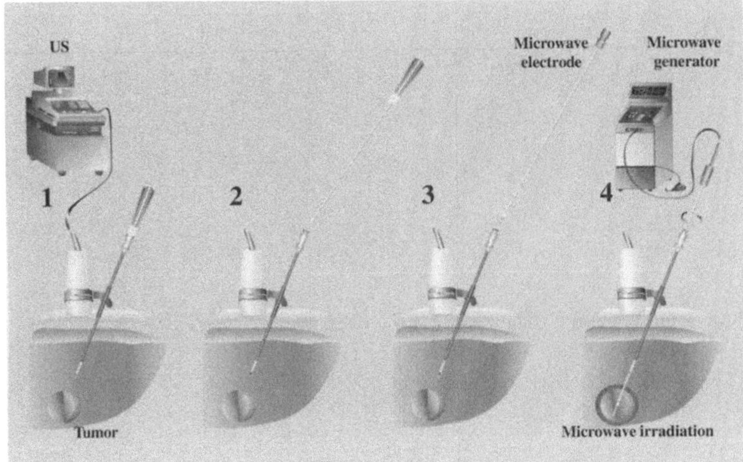

Fig. 1. The percutaneous microwave coagulation therapy (PMCT) technique. *1*, guide needle insertion; *2*, inner needle of the guide needle is removed; *3*, microwave electrode insertion; *4*, microwave irradiation

bile leakage, and cancer cell seeding when both the outer guide needle and the electrode were removed (Fig. 2).

For the purpose of acquiring reliable local control of the tumor, we attempted to induce a margin of 5mm or more of necrosis in the noncancerous tissue surrounding the tumor, that is, the treated margin (Fig. 3). At each session, two to four electrode insertions were performed for the tumor, including different sites in its proximity, and one microwave irradiation (80W for 60s) was done for each electrode insertion. We carried out dynamic computed tomography (CT) to assess the therapeutic effect 2 days after every session. The next session was made according to the findings on postsession dynamic CT. PMCT was carried out twice a week.

Follow-Up

Following discharge from the hospital, all patients were closely observed. The follow-up program included abdominal sonography every 1–2 months and abdominal dynamic CT every 3–6 months. The levels of tumor markers, α-fetoprotein (AFP) and protein induced vitamin K absence or antagonist II (PIVKAII) were measured monthly after treatment.

Patients

The 59 patients who underwent PMCT each had a single HCC measuring 2cm or less in maximal diameter (small HCC; Stage I, according to the International Union Against Cancer [4]). In all cases, histological diagnosis was confirmed by US-guided fine-needle biopsy performed at our hospital. All were diagnosed with liver cirrhosis. Clinical observation periods following treatment ranged from 12 to 80 months. All procedures were thoroughly explained to the patients, and informed consent was obtained from each.

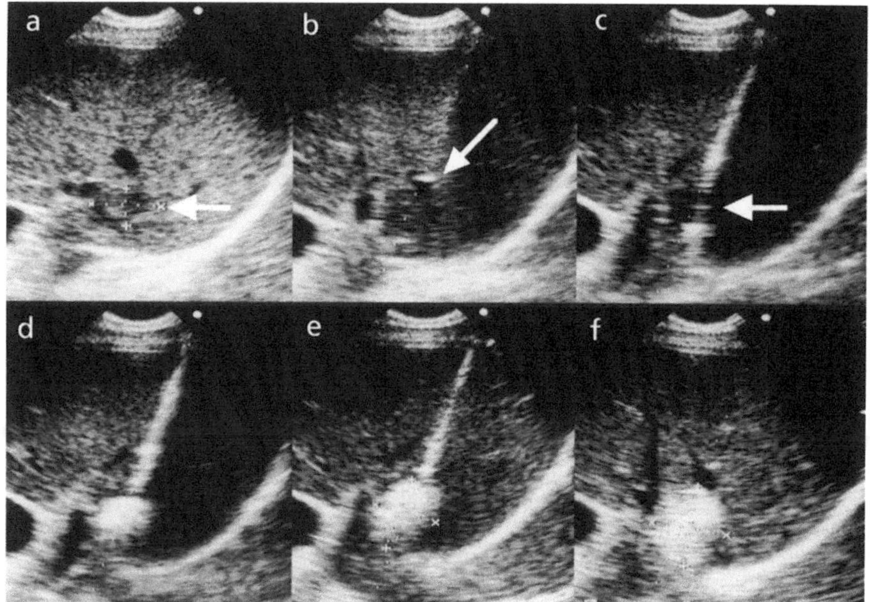

Fig. 2a–f. Ultrasonograms before, during, and after PMCT. **a** Before treatment (*white arrow*, tumor). **b** The guide needle (*white arrow*) is inserted. **c** The microwave electrode (*white arrow*) is inserted into the interior of the tumor. **d, e** The tumor is irradiated. **f** Microwave irradiation is complete

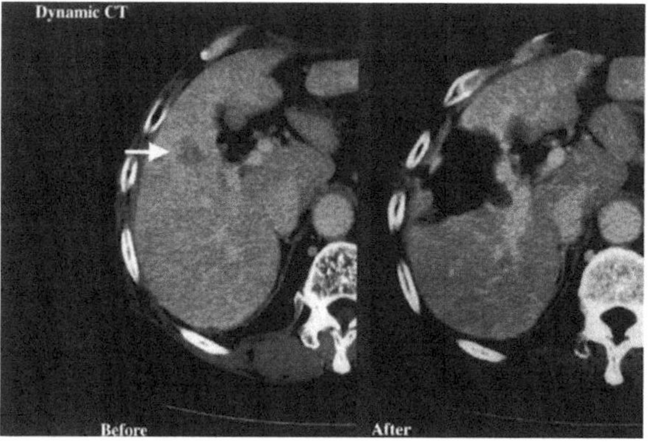

Fig. 3. Dynamic computed tomo-graphy. Before treatment (*left*). The tumor site (*white arrow*) is S5. One week after treatment (*right*). After treatment, the tumor and the surrounding area were not enhanced

Results

Treatment Efficacy

The PMCT of the tumors was completed within 1 week for all patients. One to two sessions were employed (mean, 1.6 sessions).

After three to four microwave irradiations were performed for a tumor ≤ 1.5 cm and four to six irradiations for a tumor >1.5 cm, at the greatest dimension, 55 of 59 patients showed complete necrosis of the tumor lesion with a treated margin ≥ 5 mm on dynamic CT. To obtain a treated margin ≥ 5 mm, a large number of microwave irradiations (six electrode insertions) was necessary for some patients, possibly because of the cooling effect of circulated blood.

In the other four patients, although complete necrosis of the tumor lesion was obtained, the parenchyma surrounding the tumor was still viable because PMCT could not be performed extensively as the gallbladder or large blood vessels were near the tumor.

Survival

The 5-year overall survival rate of patients with small HCC treated with PMCT was 70% and their 5-year cancer-free survival rate was 22%.

Pattern of Recurrence

Only three patients experienced a return of the lesions at the same subsegment in which the initial tumor was seen within 2 years after PMCT. There were no definite local recurrences during the follow-up period.

Adverse Effects and Complications Of PMCT

All patients complained of a slight heat sensation in the upper abdominal region during PMCT. Half the patients felt some pain during treatment, but it was not serious enough to stop the course of treatment. Local dissemination of the cancer cells along the puncture line was not encountered in any case. However, we experienced some complications, such as pleural effusion (three patients), subcapsular hematoma (one patient), and intrahepatic duct stricture (one patient).

Discussion

Percutaneous ethanol injection therapy (PEIT) is now often performed for patients with small HCCs. However, a number of reports in which the effects of PEIT were evaluated histopathologically and clinically have demonstrated that the injected ethanol did not always cause complete necrosis of the tumor [5]. We often observe viable cancer cells persisting in the extra- or intracapsular area in surgically resected or autopsy specimens after PEIT. These viable cells have the potential to cause local recurrences, as well as both intrahepatic and distant metastases, and may worsen the patient's prognosis.

To resolve these problems, we designed PMCT as a new local treatment to acquire reliable tissue coagulation. PMCT, which we formulated in this study, heats tissue by molecular vibration of dipoles, particularly of water in tissue, and induces thermal coagulation in the target area. Regardless of the presence of a fibrous capsule surrounding the tumor, microwave irradiation is most reliable in inducing tissue coagulation.

In this study, the 5-year overall survival rate of patients with small HCC treated with PMCT was relatively good, compared with that of patients treated with PEIT that were previously reported [6,7]. On the other hand, the cancer-free survival of patients treated with PMCT was not as good. However, the recurrences after PMCT were mainly observed in a different subsegment than that in which the initial nodule was seen. This result shows that PMCT has a reliable coagulation capability for the tumor area. Therefore, we consider that this reliable local control capability of PMCT may reduce intrahepatic metastases from a initial tumor or microscopic metastases adjacent to the primary tumor and improve the patient's prognosis.

This study was not a prospective randomized trial and has the potential for selection biases of treatment groups. Therefore, in assessing the therapeutic efficacy of PMCT, there is a great need for a multicenter randomized controlled trial compared with PEIT or other treatments with longer follow-up and a larger series. Based on our experience, however, we think that PMCT may be a first choice among the therapeutic modalities for small liver cancer because of its reliable therapeutic effects and low invasiveness.

References

1. Okuda K, Ohtsuki T, Obata H, Tomimatu M, Okazaki N, Hasegawa H, Nakajima Y, Ohnishi K (1985) Natural history of hepatocellular carcinoma and prognosis in relation to treatment: study of 850 patients. Cancer (Phila) 56:918–928
2. Kuroda C, Sakurai M, Monden M, Marukawa T, Hosoki T, Tokunaga K, Wakasa K, Okamura J, Kozuka T (1991) Limitation of transcatheter arterial chemoembolization using iodized oil for small hepatocellular carcinoma: a study in resected cases. Cancer (Phila) 67:81–86
3. Seki T, Wakabayashi M, Nakagawa T, Itho T, Shiro T, Kunieda K, Uchiyama S, Inoue K (1994) Ultrasonically guided percutaneous microwave coagulation therapy for small hepatocellular carcinoma. Cancer (Phila) 74:814–825
4. Sobin LH, Wittekind CH (1997) TNM classification of malignant tumors, 5th edn. Wiley-Liss, New York, pp 74–77
5. Shiina S, Tagawa K, Unuma T, Takanashi R, Yoshiura K, Komatsu Y, Hata Y (1991) Percutaneous ethanol injection therapy for hepatocellular carcinoma: a histopathologic study. Cancer (Phila) 68:1524–1530
6. Ebara M, Ohto M, Sugiura N, Kita K, Yoshikawa M, Okuda K, Kond F, Kondo Y (1990) Percutaneous ethanol injection for the treatment of small hepatocellular carcinoma: study of 95 patients. J Gastroenterol Hepatol 5:616–626
7. Toyoda H, Kumada T, Nakano S, Takeda I, Sugiyama K, Kiriyama S, Sone Y (1997) Significance of tumor vascularity as a predictor of long-term prognosis in patients with small hepatocellular carcinoma treated by percutaneous ethanol injection therapy. J Hepatol 26:1055–1062

Percutaneous Ablation of Hepatocellular Carcinoma

Tito Livraghi

Summary. Percutaneous ethanol injection (PEI) is performed under ultrasound guidance, with multiple sessions in the out-patient department or with the "single-session" technique under general anesthesia, according to the size and number of the lesions. In our patients, with Child A (293), B (149), or C (20) cirrhosis and single hepatocellular carcinoma (HCC) lesions of 5 cm or smaller, the 1-, 3-, and 5-year survival rates were 98%, 79%, and 47%, 93%, 63%, and 29%, and 64%, 12%, and 0%, respectively. In our 108 patients with larger HCC, 1-, and 3-year survival rates were 72% and 57% in single, encapsulated tumors, 73% and 42% in single infiltrating or multiple encapsulated tumors, and 46% and 0% in symptomatic or with advanced portal thrombosis tumors. PEI proved to be a safe, effective, repeatable, easy, and low-cost therapy for HCC. Survival after PEI was comparable to that after surgical resection, probably because of the balance between the greater complete ablation rate of surgery compared to the absence of early mortality and liver damage using PEI. On the basis of the PEI rationale, other ablation techniques were proposed using radio frequency, laser, or acetic acid methods, and their initial results are promising.

Key words. Hepatocellular carcinoma, Liver neoplasm therapy, Interventional procedures, Cirrhosis

Introduction

Local-regional therapies are those treatment modalities which, by the percutaneous route, allow the introduction of a damaging agent directly into the neoplastic tissue. It is understood that such therapies are indicated only for those pathologies limited to a single organ, such as hepatocellular carcinoma (HCC), and not in an advanced stage. Local-regional therapies may be based on the use of means capable of destroying the tissue chemically, such as ethyl alcohol (percutaneous ethanol injection, PEI) or acetic acid, or physically (thermally), as with laser, microwave, or radiofrequency (RF). PEI was the first therapy to be proposed [1]. On the basis of its rationale and the results obtained, the other therapies were subsequently designed [2–5]. This

Department of Radiology, Ospedale Civile, Via Cereda 23, 20059 Vimercate, Milano, Italy

chapter considers mainly PEI, which is the most diffused and codified, and RF therapy, whose recent results indicate a wide development.

Percutaneous Ethanol Injection

PEI, in the treatment of hepatic tumors, was conceived independently at the University of Chiba in Japan and at the Vimercate Hospital (Milan) in Italy. The first paper in an international journal appeared in 1986 [1].

Procedure

PEI is performed in multiple sessions in an ambulatory regimen (conventional technique) [6] or, when the tumor is advanced, in a single session under general anesthesia with the patient hospitalized [7]. The former technique is generally used for single HCC less than 4–5 cm in diameter or for multiple HCC with two to three nodules less than 3 cm in diameter. The latter technique is adopted for more advanced HCC, single or multiple, that do not occupy more than 30% of the hepatic volume and with no neoplastic thrombosis in the main portal branches or in the hepatic veins. Both techniques can be repeated in the case of local recurrences or new lesions.

The modalities of the treatment may also depend on the purpose, that is, to obtain a complete response or only for a palliative result. Complete response, that is, complete necrosis, is sought when the HCC is focal, without intrahepatic metastases or portal infiltration. In such a case, if neoplastic tissue is still present at the control of therapeutic efficacy after the treatment, additional sessions are carried out until the possible attainment of complete necrosis (Fig. 1). Instead, when the presentation of the HCC generally excludes the possibility of reaching a complete response, that is, in the infiltrating form, it is sufficient to attain a substantial necrosis that determines a temporary arrest of neoplastic growth. PEI can also be used for the treatment of neoplastic portal thrombosis, when the thrombus is segmental or subsegmental, to arrest progression toward the main branches [8].

Evaluation of Therapeutic Efficacy

To evaluate the therapeutic response, as imaging modalities we use ultrasonography (US) color-Doppler with echo enhancers (Levovist, Schering, Berlin, Germany), and spiral computed tomography (CT) with biphasic technique (4 ml/s, 25 and 60 s after the injection of contrast medium). If the areas of tissue still viable are very small, beyond the present powers of resolution, they obviously are not recognizable on the images at the end of the treatment. However, they will be easily identified at successive examinations as zones of enhancement at CT. The response is considered complete when CT scan shows the total disappearance of enhancement within the tumor and when the same picture is confirmed at scans performed at successive controls.

As tumor markers, we use alpha-feto-protein (AFP) and des-γ-carboxy prothrombin (DCP), which are often complementary [9]. In reality, particularly when the HCC is relatively small, the markers often are not pathological. When the imaging

Fig. 1. a Enhanced CT scan shows an encapsulated hepatocellular carcinoma (HCC), 4.8 cm in size, 1 month after single-session percutaneous ethanol injection (PEI). Only a partial response was obtained because a small hypervascularized rounded area remained inside the tumor. **b** After two sessions of conventional PEI targeted on the residual neoplastic area, on imaging a complete response was achieved

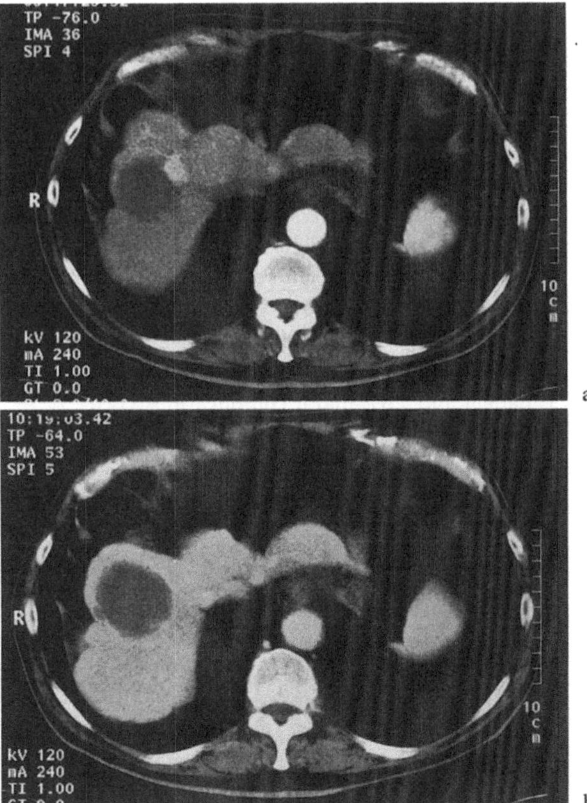

techniques show a complete response not followed by an evident reduction in AFP or DCP levels, it means that neoplastic tissue which is not detected or not yet detectable is growing elsewhere. Moreover, an increase in levels during controls always suggests a local recurrence or the appearance of new lesions. The control with US, CT, and serum assay of tumor markers is carried out for a month after treatment and then every 4–6 months.

Complications

Conventional Treatment

No death occurred in 1623 patients treated with conventional PEI and collected from different series [6]. A recent multicenter study on 1066 patients reported 1 death (0.09%) from hemoperitoneum and subsequent hepatic coma [10]. Another death caused by a massive area of hepatic necrosis distant from the site of injection of ethanol and to myocardial infarction was described in a case report; however, no direct relation was shown between the two pathologies [11]. Major complications are rare, occurring in 1.3%–3.2% of cases, and are generally treated in a conservative manner [6,10].

Single-Session Treatment

The use of greater volumes of ethanol per session determines a higher complication rate. During the first days of treatment there is a significant increase in transaminases, bilirubin, D-dimer, and white blood cells and a reduction in fibrinogen, haptoglobin, hemoglobin, platelets, and red blood cells. Such modifications, which normalize within 2 weeks, are caused by necrosis of the neoplastic and perineoplastic tissue, diffuse intra- and peritumoral microthrombosis, and hemolysis. In our series of 111 treatments, there was 1 death (0.7%) due to bleeding of esophageal varices in a Child's C patient and 4.6% major complications [12].

Results

Some long-term survival curves have been published [13–15]. Survival at 5 years of these series was respectively 51%, 48%, and 43%. A multicenter Italian study enrolled 746 patients [6]. In Child's A patients ($n = 293$), B ($n = 149$), or C ($n = 20$) with single HCC less than 5 cm in diameter, survival at 1, 3, and 5 years was respectively 98%, 79%, and 47%, 93%, 63%, and 29%, and 64%, 12%, and 0%. In Child's A patients with multiple HCC ($n = 121$), survival was 94%, 68%, and 36%. As regards HCC greater than 5 cm in diameter, a study of 108 patients reported the following results: survival at 3 years of patients with encapsulated HCC measuring 5–8.5 cm in diameter was 57%; with infiltrating HCC measuring 5–10 cm or multiple HCC, 42%; and with advanced HCC, that is, already symptomatic or with lobar portal thrombosis, 0% [12].

The main cause of death in Child's A patients was progression of the neoplastic disease mainly because of the appearance of new lesions; in Child's C patients it was hepatic insufficiency. The incidence of appearance of new lesions at 5 years in the group of patients from the University of Chiba was 87%, in the Shiina group 64%, and in the Tanikawa group about 100%. In our study, the overall incidence was 87%, 74% in patients with single HCC, and 98% in patients with multiple HCC. The incidence of local recurrences was 4%, 7%, and 17%, according to the authors [6,13,14].

Discussion

The following points constitute the rationale to resort to PEI.

1. The expansive type of HCC initially shows a regional growth, so that a local therapy such as PEI can be used.

2. US screening of a cirrhotic population identifies HCC at an early stage, when the tumor is still small. In a study by Oka et al. [16], most of the patients (82%) had an HCC less than 5 cm in diameter.

3. Ethanol shows a selective diffusion in HCC, owing to the tumor's soft consistency with respect to surrounding cirrhotic tissue and its hypervascularity.

4. Alcoholization does not have the disadvantage of loss or important damage of nonneoplastic parenchyma. In the series of Shiina et al. [17], histological examination of resected pieces did not reveal important alterations of the peritumoral tissue. In contrast, it is likely that the loss of healthy tissue from a multisegmentary resection or parenchymal damage following a massive transaarterial chemoembolization determines deterioration of hepatic function and an anticipation of terminal insufficiency [18,19].

5. PEI is a low-risk method. In series published up to now, the mortality rate has been insignificant, and the highest complication rate is 3.2%, with most complications treated in a conservative manner. The absence of mortality with conventional PEI is in marked contrast with the perioperative mortality from surgery, which even though much lower than in the past, is a factor to take into consideration, especially in centers with little experience. Centers with extensive experience report a mortality rate of 1.4%–11% and a complication rate as high as 58% [6]. In this regard, it should be remembered that patients selected by US screening are asymptomatic and that, even if untreated, have a life expectancy of more than 1 year [20].

6. PEI can be easily repeated when new lesions appear, as happens in most patients within 5 years. The incidence of appearance of new lesions in surgical series varies from 67% to 100% [6]. In our series treated with PEI, it was 65%–98%. The finding, which should always be taken into consideration whenever a choice of treatment must be made, can be ascribed to the multicentric nature of HCC in patients with chronic hepatitis [21]. This means that the first lesion evidenced at US is usually the prelude to others and that surgery, even if radical on resected lesions, is generally only palliative as regards the natural history of the disease. At the University of Chiba, the incidence of appearance of new lesions in two groups of patients comparably treated with surgery and PEI was identical [22]. Because this finding reflects the natural history of the disease, the patient should be followed frequently so that new lesions can be treated as they form and are still small. In this regard, an advantage of PEI is that the patient is followed by the same physician in the diagnostic as well as therapeutic phase. Moreover, it is now possible with single-session PEI to also further interfere with the course of the disease in some patients who would not have benefited from conventional PEI.

7. The low cost, easy availability of the necessary material, and the simplicity of the technique make it possible to perform PEI anywhere, so that many hospitals, even peripheral, can apply it without resorting to a referral center. The patients are generally treated on an outpatient basis, and most of them can carry on a normal daily life. The materials (needle, syringe, alcohol) costs very little and are readily available. In Italy, the cost of one PEI cycle is about $1 000, that of orthotopic liver transplantation (OLT) about $125 000, and of a partial hepatectomy about $30 000. In Japan, Kotoh et al. [23] reported an average cost of $759 for outpatient PEI and $27 105 for resection. Because the annual number of patients who will develop the disease is about

20 000–25 000 in Japan and about 12 000 in Italy [6], the problem of costs is not of secondary importance.

8. The local therapeutic efficacy of PEI is rather high. Histopathological studies of resected pieces were carried out particularly in the initial period of treatment with PEI. In our experience, 6 of 8 lesions (75%) showed complete necrosis and 2 of 8 showed 90% necrosis. In a study aimed at the problem, Shiina et al. [17] demonstrated complete necrosis in 16 of 23 lesions (69.5%), 90% necrosis in 6 lesions, and 70% necrosis in 1 lesion. The study showed that the viable tissue was present in small satellite nodules around the main lesions, along the lesion margins, or in correspondence to septa.

9. The long-term results with PEI are good. No controlled studies have reported on PEI compared to no treatment, but the same is true for surgery. It was apparent from the beginning that PEI was an efficacious treatment without risks, so that it was not considered ethical to create an arm of untreated patients. Comparisons with no treatment are consequently based only on historical data. Of two studies on untreated patients with comparable disease, the first on 27 patients reported a 5-year survival of 0% and the second, on 73 patients, of 11% [13,19]. Recently, a case-control study in Child's A patients with HCC less than 4 cm in diameter statistically confirmed the validity of PEI compared to no treatment, with survival at 3 years of 71% and 21%, respectively [24]. In a comparative study based on historical data, the mean overall survival at 5 years for 628 patients with lesions less than 5 cm and compensated cirrhosis treated with PEI was 48%, whereas that of 1 272 resected patients with a similar presentation was 49% [6]. Such data were recently confirmed by a multicentric Japanese study in which survival at 5 years of 445 resected patients was 54% and of 110 patients treated with PEI was 53% [25]. The substantial comparability can probably be attributed to a balance between advantages and disadvantages of the two therapies: the greater percentage of complete ablation with resection, in favor of surgery; and the absence of perioperative mortality (which on average is 7% in the most important surgical series), the absence of nonneoplastic tissue loss, the insufficient evaluation of prognostic factors in resected patients, and the downstaging of imaging examinations, in favor of PEI.

In conclusion, the large number of patients enrolled in US screening programs has created a demand for an effective, safe, repeatable, and economic treatment that can be made available in many centers. PEI substantially satisfies all such requisites. In the absence of randomized studies and on the basis of reported results, PEI is indicated as the treatment of choice for most patients enrolled by US screening, excluding those who are candidates for OLT and for surgical resection. Unfortunately, the former is available only for very few patients. As regards the indications for surgery, the Liver Cancer Study Group of Japan has reported factors predictive for a long-term prognosis [26]. At multivariate analysis, the most important predictive factors, in decreasing order, were AFP level, tumor size, number of lesions, age of the patient, stage of cirrhosis, margins of resection, and portal thrombosis. Univariate analysis showed capsular infiltration, tumor extent, and Edmondson–Stainer classification to be the most important. Nevertheless, although there is a certain perioperative mortality and discrete morbidity with surgery, so that the patients should be selected very carefully to eliminate every factor that may affect the long-term results, PEI is rarely accompanied by complications and thus patient selection can be less restricted.

In our opinion, PEI is therefore indicated in patients who are (1) not candidates for OLT; (2) not resectable; (3a) resectable but presenting with one of the negative prognostic factors of the aforementioned multivariate analysis (high AFP, age over 70 years, multinodularity, Child's B disease, vascular infiltration); or (3b) resectable with only enucleation, in that such surgery does not remove eventual peritumoral satellites (which is also a limitation of PEI). In fact, patients subjected to enucleation, in addition to having a significantly shorter survival than those who undergo segmentectomy, also have a shorter survival than that obtained with PEI [27]. However, it is still debated whether a complex or multisegmentary resection is an appropriate therapy for a small HCC. In addition, the surgical center should assure a low perioperative mortality, at least 3% or less. In practice, most patients could be managed as follows: early identification of the HCC by means of US screening, treatment with PEI, follow-up with imaging methods and tumor markers, and treatment of new lesions with PEI.

Thermoablation with Radio Frequency

Principles

The treatment of thermoablation with RF exploits the conversion of the energy of an electromagnetic wave into heat. A generator is used that converts normal energy supplied by an electric alternating current of 90 Hz into the RF band of 500 kHz. The current is linked to an active electrode in the form of a needle, which is inserted into the tumor so that the body becomes part of the electric circuit, and is dispersed with a passive electrode in the form of a plate, which is applied to the skin of the patient. In this way, a resistive type of heating is produced, particularly around the exposed point of the needle electrode, caused by ionic agitation of the tissue electrolytes that follow the change in direction of the alternating current. Heat is generated by means of the impedance (resistance) that the surrounding tissue opposes to the flow of current, so that heat is not generated at the tip of the electrode but within the tissue. The heat produced is given by the difference between the heat generated around the extremity of the electrode and dispersed heat, whose entity depends on the conductivity of the tissue and dissipation by convection due to blood circulation.

When a conventional RF technique is used, a reproducible area of necrosis is obtained, but it does not exceed 1.6 cm in diameter [28]. The difficulty in reaching greater dimensions is caused by carbonization of the tissue, which, being a poor conductor, increases impedance and self-limits propagation of the current. Therefore, in tumors of greater volume, more insertions are necessary. Nevertheless, it was observed that correct positioning of the electrodes was often technically difficult, with the result that the desired volume and form of necrosis was rarely obtained. To overcome such difficulties, other techniques have been proposed: bipolar, multipolar, or unipolar with simultaneous instillation of a saline solution to increase the extension of the active surface [29]. All these techniques, although succeeding in obtaining wider areas of necrosis, at the same time presented limitations and difficulties that made their use unsatisfactory.

Two other technological advances have been recently proposed. The first uses an expandable electrode 1.9 mm in diameter, which, once positioned in the tumor, opens out into three or four hooks around the target like an umbrella. This technique determines a reproducible area of necrosis about 3 cm in diameter [30]. The second method utilizes a cold perfusion electrode with a diameter of 1.2 mm and the tip exposed for 2–4 cm [31,32]. As already stated, during the application of conventional RF, the highest temperatures are reached in strict proximity of the electrode tip, to then rapidly diminish near the periphery. The carbonization that occurs above 100°C around the tip is the main factor that limits the amount of power to be applied. Starting therefore from the hypothesis that to obtain a greater diameter of necrosis it is necessary to diminish the temperature in the proximity of the electrode surface, perfusion or cold-tip electrodes were developed. By avoiding early increments of impedance linked to carbonization, such electrodes permit application of a greater power with respect to conventional electrodes (70–75 W compared to 20–30 W). To obtain cooling, a physiological solution brought to 2°–5°C is circulated within two coaxial lumens situated in the electrode. In a preliminary study, Goldberg et al. [31] obtained, with a single insertion of a perfusion monopolar electrode with 3 cm of the tip exposed, an area of coagulative necrosis of 2.4 cm in diameter in the in vivo liver of animals. A recently constructed electrode with three tips, permitting a higher current deposition, permits even greater areas of necrosis.

Technique

Therapy with RF does not differ substantially from that of PEI as regards the technique of introduction, the investigations and parameters used to evaluate therapeutic efficacy, and their cadence. In our center, patients are always hospitalized for 2 days. Because the procedure may be painful, it is performed under sedation when one or at the most two insertions are foreseen, or under general anesthesia with tracheal intubation when a greater number is planned. The therapy plan foresees the completion of therapy in only one session, with an eventual retreatment after the first control of therapeutic efficacy.

We use a generator capable of producing 200 W of power (CC1, Radionics, Burlington, MA, USA) and of monitoring the temperature at the electrode tip, the impedance, and the intensity (maximum, 2000 mA). The length of the exposed tip, which can vary from 2 to 4 cm, is chosen as a function of the size of the desired ablation volume, which depends in turn on the size of the tumor. The maximum milliamperage is maintained as such until the end of the insertion for 10–12 min. During the deposition of energy, a hyperechoic spot forms around the electrode because of vaporization and intratissue cavitation and tends to progressively widen during the treatment. At the same time numerous hyperechogenic microbubbles of vapor are visible along the hepatic veins.

Indications

As regards patients treated with PEI, the indications for HCC less than 3 cm in diameter are the same, with the exception of tumors located in a site considered at risk for RF (hepatic hilum; difficult approach). There are still no precise indications as regards larger HCC. Theoretically, at the beginning of the experience, the diameter of expected tissue necrosis was 2.4 cm, that is, that obtained in the liver of animals with the tip exposed for 3 cm [31]. Unexpectedly, it was observed that in an HCC 3 cm in diameter the area and shape of the necrosis reproduced that of the original tumor like a mold. Such an effect was designated the "oven effect," in that it was believed that the surrounding cirrhotic tissue, for its high fibrotic component, was a poor conductor and thus functioned as an insulating material, allowing a higher deposition of energy within the neoplastic tissue [33].

Results

Two studies have been published on the treatment of HCC with RF. The first was carried out using a hooked expandable electrode on 23 patients with HCC up to 3.5 cm in diameter. With an average of 1.4 sessions, a complete response was reported in all the tumors. No complications were observed [30].

The second was a controlled prospective study that compared PEI and RF on 86 patients with 112 HCC measuring up to 3 cm in diameter. A complete response was reached in 90.3% with RF and in 80.0% with PEI. Such results were obtained with an average of 1.2 sessions for RF and 4.8 sessions for PEI. However, there were more complications with RF, that is, one severe (hemothorax that required drainage) and four minor, compared to none with PEI [33]. On the basis of such findings, we have abandoned PEI as a therapy of tumors of this size, except for lesions considered at risk for the site. Benefiting from "the oven effect," preliminary results in large HCC are interesting (Fig. 2). The side effects caused by the large amount of ethanol administered with PEI in a single session were not observed. Consequently, a comparative study in more advanced HCC is ongoing.

Conclusions

PEI, conceived to treat inoperable patients, has increasingly gained popularity, so that it is today often preferred to resection. Its easy execution, low cost, low incidence of complications, the possibility of repeating it on new lesions, and finally results similar to those obtained with surgery are the main factors of its success. The wide diffusion of PEI has opened a debate with surgeons, who in the course of the last years have improved resection and postoperative techniques. In the absence of randomized studies, it is and will be very difficult to find consensual accord on the indications of the respective therapies. At the moment, the only course is to extrapolate from retrospective comparative studies, although affected by bias, and from studies on prognostic factors at least the unequivocal information that can prevent useless or even

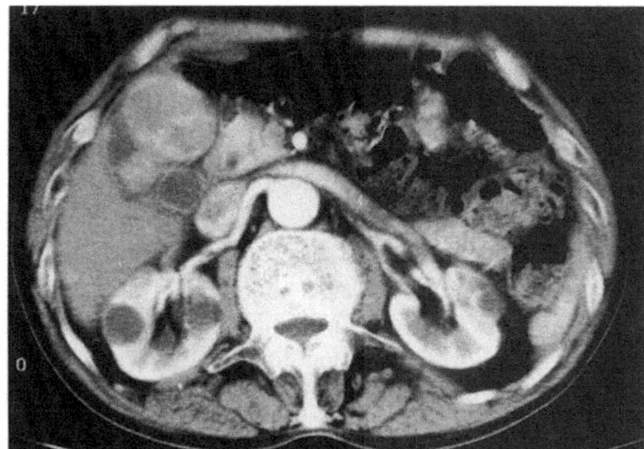

a

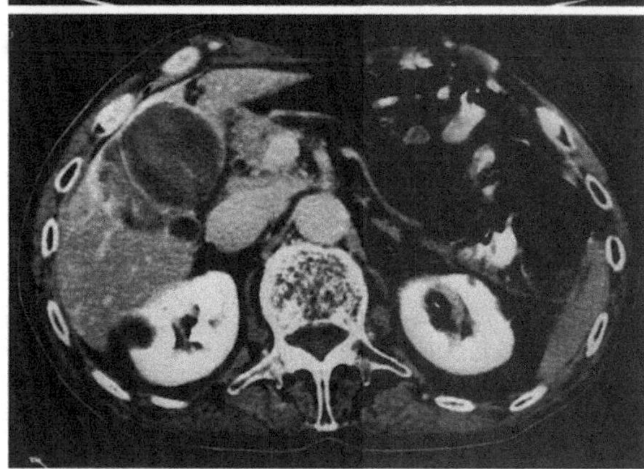

b

Fig. 2. a Enhanced CT scan shows an encapsulated HCC, 5.8 cm in size, located near the gallbladder, before radiofrequency ablation. **b** The HCC after therapy appeared completely hypodense and devoid of enhancement because of destruction of the vascular supply. On imaging, a complete response was obtained

damaging therapies. In short, candidates for surgery are those patients who do not present one of the aforementioned negative prognostic factors, in whom an anatomical resection is possible, and in whom the loss of nonneoplastic tissue is proportional to the size of the tumor. As regards other percutaneous ablative therapies, none of them has changed the rationale on which treatment with PEI is based. From these, we await only an increased percentage of complete response, while still maintaining the safety of PEI.

References

1. Livraghi T, Festi D, Monti F, Salmi A, Vettori C (1986) US-guided percutaneous alcohol injection of small hepatic and abdominal tumors. Radiology 161:309–312
2. Ohnishi K, Ohyama M, Ito S, Fujiara K (1994) Ultrasound guided intratumor injection of acetic acid for the treatment of small hepatocellular carcinoma. Radiology 193: 747–752

3. Masters A, Steger AC, Lees WR (1992) Interstitial laser hyperthermia: a new approach for treating liver metastases. Br J Cancer 66:518–522

4. Rossi S, Fornari F, Buscarini L (1993) Percutaneous ultrasound guided radiofrequency electrocautery for the treatment of small hepatocellular carcinoma. J Intervent Radiol 8:97–103

5. Murakami R, Yoshimatsu S, Yamashita Y, Matsukawa T, Takahashi M, Sagara K (1995) Treatment of hepatocellular carcinoma: value of percutaneous microwave coagulation. AJR 164:1159–1164

6. Livraghi T, Giorgio A, Marin G, Salmi A, de Sio I, Bolondi L, Pompili M, Brunello F, Lazzaroni S, Torzilli G, Zucchi A (1995) Hepatocellular carcinoma and cirrhosis in 746 patients: long-term results of percutaneous ethanol injection. Radiology 197: 101–108

7. Livraghi T, Vettori C, Torzilli G, Lazzaroni S, Pellicanò S, Ravasi S (1993) Percutaneous ethanol injection of hepatic tumors: single session therapy under general anesthesia. AJR 160:1065–1069

8. Livraghi T, Grigioni W, Mazziotti A, Sangalli G, Vettori C (1990) Percutaneous ethanol injection of portal thrombosis in hepatocellular carcinoma: a new possible treatment. Tumori 76:394–397

9. Shimada M, Takenaka K, Fujiwara Y, Gion T, Kajiyama K, Maeda T, Shirabe K, Sugimachi K (1996) Des-gamma-carboxy prothrombin and AFP positive status as a new prognostic indicator after hepatic resection for hepatocellular carcinoma. Cancer (Phila) 78:2094–2100

10. Di Stasi M, Buscarini T, Livraghi T, Giorgio A, Salmi A, De Sio I, Brunello F, Solmi L, Caturelli E, Magnolfi F, Caremani M, Filice C (1997) Percutaneous ethanol injection in the treatment of hepatocellular carcinoma. Scand J Gastroenterol 32:1168–1173

11. Taavitsainen M, Vehmas T, Kauppila R (1993) Fatal liver necrosis following percutaneous ethanol injection for hepatocellular carcinoma. Abdom Imaging 18:357–359

12. Livraghi T, Benedini V, Lazzaroni S, Meloni F, Torzilli G, Vettori C (1998) Long-term results of single session PEI in patients with large hepatocellular carcinoma. Cancer (Phila) 83:48–57

13. Ebara M, Otho M, Sugiura N, Okuda K, Kondo F, Kondo K (1990) Percutaneous ethanol injection for the treatment of small hepatocellular carcinoma: study of 95 patients. J Gastroenterol Hepatol 5:616–626

14. Shiina S, Tagawa K, Niwa Y, Unuma T, Komatsu Y, Yoshiura K, Hamada E, Takahasi M, Shiratori Y, Terano A, Omata M, Kawauchi N, Inoue H (1993) Percutaneous ethanol injection therapy for hepatocellular carcinoma: results in 146 patients. AJR 160: 1023–1028

15. Tanikawa K (1992) Multidisciplinary treatment of hepatocellular carcinoma. In: Tobe T, Kameda H (eds) Primary liver cancer in Japan. Springer-Verlag, Tokyo, pp 327–334

16. Oka H, Kurioka N, Kim K, Kanno T, Kuroki T, Mizoguchi Y, Kobayashi K (1990) Prospective study of early detection of hepatocellular carcinoma in patients with cirrhosis. Hepatology 12:680–687

17. Shiina S, Tagawa K, Unuma T, Takanashi R, Yoshiura K, Komatsu Y, Hata Y, Niwa Y, Shiratori Y, Terano A, Sugimoto T (1991) Percutaneous ethanol injection therapy for hepatocellular carcinoma: a histopathologic study. Cancer (Phila) 68:1524–1530

18. Yamashita Y, Torashima M, Ognuni T, Yamamoto A, Harada M, Miyazaki T, Takahashi M (1993) Liver parenchymal changes after transcatheter arterial embolization therapy for hepatoma. CT evaluation. Abdom Imaging 18:352–356

19. Groupe d'Etude et de Traitement du Carcinome Hepatocellulaire (1995) A comparison of lipiodol chemoembolization and conservative treatment for unresectable hepatocellular carcinoma. N Engl J Med 332:1256–1261

20. Livraghi T, Bolondi L, Buscarini L, Cottone M, Mazziotti A, Morabito A, Torzilli G (1995) No treatment, resection and ethanol injection in hepatocellular carcinoma: a retrospective analysis of survival in 391 cirrhotic patients. J Hepatol 22:522–526
21. Sheu JC, Huang GT, Chou HC (1993) Multiple hepatocellular carcinomas at the early stage have different clonality. Gastroenterology 105:1471–1476
22. Okuda K (1993) Intratumor ethanol injection. J Surg Oncol 3(suppl):97–99
23. Kotoh K, Sakai H, Sakamoto S, Nakayama S, Satoh M, Morotomi I, Nawata H (1994) The effect of percutaneous ethanol injection therapy on small solitary hepatocellular carcinoma is comparable to that of hepatectomy. Am J Gastroenterol 89:194–198
24. Orlando A, Cottone M, Virdone R, Parisi P, Maringhini A, Caltagirone M, Simonetti R, Pagliaro L (1997) Treatment of small hepatocellular carcinoma associated with cirrhosis by percutaneous ethanol injection. Scand J Gastroenterol 32:598–603
25. Ryu M, Shimamura Y, Kinoshita T, Konishi M, Kawano N, Iwasaki M, Furuse J, Yoshino M, Moriyama N, Sugita M (1997) Therapeutic results of resection, TAE and PEI in 3 225 patients with hepatocellular carcinoma: a retrospective multicenter study. Jpn J Clin Oncol 27:251–257
26. The Liver Cancer Study Group of Japan (1994) Predictive factors for long-term prognosis after partial hepatectomy for patients with hepatocellular carcinoma. Cancer (Phila) 74:2772–2780
27. Takayama T, Makuuchi M (1997) Surgical resection. In: Livraghi T, Makuuchi M, Buscarini L (eds) Diagnosis and treatment of hepatocellular carcinoma. Greenwich Medical Media, London, pp 279–286
28. Goldberg SN, Gazelle GS, Dawson SL, Mueller PR, Rittman W, Rosenthal DI (1995) Radiofrequency tissue ablation using multiprobe arrays: greater tissue destruction than multiple probes operating alone. Acad Radiol 2:670–674
29. Livraghi T, Goldberg SN, Monti F (1997) Saline-enhanced radiofrequency tissue ablation in the treatment of liver metastases. Radiology 202:205–210
30. Rossi S, Buscarini E, Garbagnati F (1988) Percutaneous treatment of small hepatic tumors by an expandable RF needle electrode. AJR 170:1015–1022
31. Goldberg SN, Gazelle GS, Solbiati L, Rittman WJ, Mueller PR (1996) Radiofrequency tissue ablation: increased lesion diameter with a perfusion electrode. Acad Radiol 3:636–644
32. Solbiati L, Goldberg SN, Ierace T, Livraghi T, Mueller PR, Gazelle GS (1997) Radiofrequency ablation of hepatic metastases with cooled-tip electrodes: results in 33 patients. Radiology 205:367–373
33. Livraghi T, Goldberg SN, Lazzaroni S, Meloni F, Solbiati L, Gazelle GS (1999) Radiofrequency ablation vs. ethanol injection in the treatment of small hepatocellular carcinoma. Radiology 210:655–661

Treatment with Subsegmental Transcatheter Arterial Embolization for Hepatocellular Carcinoma: Prognosis, Recurrence, and Effect on Liver Function

YUKIHIRO SHIROTA[1], TARO YAMASHITA[1], SHUICHI TERASAKI[1], EIKI MATSUSHITA[1], TAKESHI URABE[1], SHUICHI KANEKO[1], KENICHI KOBAYASHI[1], and OSAMU MATSUI[2]

Summary. Forty-three patients with hepatocellular carcinomas (HCCs) who had undergone subsegmental transcatheter arterial embolization (sTAE) as initial treatment were studied retrospectively to evaluate the prognosis, recurrence, and effect of sTAE on liver function. Frequent recurrences were observed (disease-free survival rates were 51.2% at 1 year and 7.7% at 3 years), and in the recurrent nodules, 66.4% were distant recurrences. No significant difference was observed in the periods of distant recurrence compared with local recurrence, and also in the periods of distant recurrence with and without local recurrence, implying that strict control of the primary lesion did not prevent distant recurrence. Concerning the effect of sTAE on liver function, ALT and LDH were significantly elevated and albumin was significantly reduced after sTAE ($p = 0.002$, < 0.0001, and $= 0.0009$, respectively). But 4 weeks after sTAE, all these levels recovered to their previous values. Moreover transient hepatic reserve reduction after sTAE did not affect the prognosis. In conclusion, for HCCs with such levels of recurrence, strict follow-up and repeat treatments with minimum damage to the hepatic reserve are essential. sTAE is an appropriate and reasonable treatment for such HCCs because of low levels of damage to the hepatic reserve and the possibility of repeat operations. Using sTAE as the main treatment against HCC, survival rates of more than 70% at 3 years were achieved.

Key words. sTAE, HCC, Recurrence, Prognosis, Liver function

Introduction

Hepatocellular carcinoma (HCC) is one of the most common malignant tumors around the world. With advances in imaging modalities and the establishment of criteria for groups at high risk for HCC [1,2], the number of candidates for effective local treatments such as surgical treatment have increased. However, because of associated liver cirrhosis and occasional multicentricity, many cases are inoperable. Therefore, transcatheter arterial embolization (TAE) plays an important role in the treatment of

[1] First Department of Internal Medicine and [2] Department of Radiology, Kanazawa University, 13-1 Takara-Machi, Kanazawa, Ishikawa, Japan

HCCs and has been widely carried out as a nonsurgical treatment [3–7]. Whether TAE improves the prognosis of patients with HCC has been controversial [8–13]. One main reason for this controversy is damage to the hepatic reserve after TAE. Another is the high frequency of recurrence after TAE treatment. Subsegmental TAE (sTAE) is performed with a microcatheter inserted into more distal branches of the subsegmental artery of the liver [14], and the HCC, along with the surrounding subsegment, is embolized [14–17].

We performed a retrospective study to analyze the survival rate, recurrence, and the effect on liver function in patients undergoing sTAE as the initial treatment for HCC to elucidate its usefulness.

Materials and Methods

Sixty-two patients with HCC(s) underwent sTAE as initial treatment. The therapeutic effects of sTAE were evaluated and classified into two groups by the imaging characteristics of the nodules. Patients in whom nodules in which the Lipiodol accumulation pattern was complete [18] on CT 1 week after treatment with no vascular lesion detected by dynamic contrast-enhanced CT 1 month after treatment were classified as the complete response group (CR). Others who did not satisfy these conditions were classified as the partial response group (PR).

In 62 patients receiving sTAE as initial therapy, 38 were classified in the CR group and 24 were classified in the PR group. Of the 24 PR patients, 18 underwent percutaneous ethanol injection therapy (PEIT) and 1 patient underwent chemotherapy. No additional treatment was performed in 5 patients because of nonvisualization on ultrasonography or contraindications for PEIT such as the existence of ascites. Overall, 43 patients underwent sTAE as initial therapy, and these were investigated in the following studies. Each procedure was followed up with dynamic contrast-enhanced CT or MRI at intervals of 3–6 months after the initial treatment. The effect of sTAE on liver function was evaluated by changes in serum ALT, LDH, bilirubin, and albumin levels at, 1, 2, and 4 weeks after sTAE treatment compared to the values before treatment.

Results

Patient and Tumor Characteristics of 43 Patients Treated With sTAE as
Initial Therapy

The average age of patients was 64.2 years, and the number of men and women was 27 and 16. Only HBsAg was positive in 5 patients, only HCV-Ab was positive in 36 patients, and both viral markers were positive in 2 patients. The clinical stage was stage I in 21 patients, II in 18, and III in 4. In terms of tumor characteristics, 13 patients were stage I, 18 were stage II, 4 were stage III, and 8 were stage IV. Twenty-nine patients had a single tumor and 14 had multiple tumors. The size of the main tumor was less than 2 cm in 20 patients, 2–4 cm in 16, and more than 4 cm in 7.

Cumulative and Disease-Free Survival Curves for 43 Patients

Cumulative survival rates were 95.3%, 71.8%, and 47.9% at 1, 3, and 5 years, respectively, but frequent recurrences were observed after sTAE. Disease-free survival rates were 51.2% and 7.7% at 1 and 3 years, respectively. The discrepancy between these two survival curves indicates that recurrence after sTAE does not directly result in poor prognosis.

Recurrence after sTAE

Distant recurrence without local recurrence was observed in 14 patients, and both local and distant recurrence were observed in 11 patients. Thus, distant recurrence occurred in 25 patients (58.2%). Among the 107 recurrent nodules, 71 nodules (66.4%) were observed distant from the primary lesions. Of these distant recurrences, 73.2% were observed in different subsegments of the liver from the primary tumor. These results show that after sTAE, distant recurrences were more frequently observed than local recurrences and that strict control of local recurrence alone was not enough to improve prognosis.

Survival Curves of Patients with Local and Distant Recurrence

To elucidate the characteristics of distant recurrences frequently observed after sTAE, survival curves of patients with local and distant recurrences were analyzed. In 85.7% of patients, distant recurrences occurred within 2 years of sTAE treatment, and there was no significant difference compared with local recurrences. This result indicates that distant recurrence also occurs in the period soon after sTAE.

Distant Recurrence-Free Survival Curves With or Without Local Recurrence

Distant recurrence-free survival curves with or without local recurrence were calculated to elucidate whether strict control of the primary lesion resulted in the reduction of distant recurrence. There was no significant difference in distant recurrence-free survival curves between patients with or without local recurrence. Thus, strict control of the primary lesion does not reduce distant recurrence.

Prediction of Distant Recurrence

Stepwise regression was performed to show which factors affect distant recurrence. The factors tested were age, sex, clinical stage, number of primary HCCs, diameter of the main HCC, number of satellite nodules, value of AFP before sTAE, number of local recurrences, and the number of times sTAE was carried out. Selected subjects were the number of primary HCCs and sex, but low r values (0.509) indicated no significant correlation between these factors and distant recurrence. This result means that it is difficult to predict distant recurrence from these factors.

Effect of sTAE on Liver Function

The effect of sTAE on liver function was analyzed by the observation of changes in ALT, LDH, albumin, and bilirubin values before and after sTAE. ALT and LDH were transiently elevated 1 week after sTAE and significantly ($p = 0.002$, and < 0.0001, respectively) recovered 2 weeks later. Albumin was significantly ($p = 0.0009$) reduced after sTAE and recovered 4 weeks after sTAE. No statistically significant change was observed in bilirubin. The changes in liver function after sTAE were transient.

Cumulative Survival Curves in Patients with Different Changes of Albumin and Bilirubin after sTAE

To elucidate whether transient reduction of hepatic reserve affects the prognosis, the prognosis was analyzed in two groups in which the changes of albumin or bilirubin after sTAE were more or less than 0.5 (g/dl or mg/dl, respectively). There was no significant difference between the prognoses of these two groups both for albumin and bilirubin. These results indicate that transient hepatic reserve reduction after sTAE does not affect the prognosis.

Conclusion

More than 65% of recurrent nodules after sTAE occurred distant from the primary lesion in the early period, almost the same value as for local recurrence. Thus, strict control of the primary lesion did not prevent distant recurrence. For HCCs with such levels of recurrence, strict follow up and repeat treatments with minimum damage to the hepatic reserve are essential. sTAE is an appropriate and reasonable treatment for such HCCs because of low levels of damage to the hepatic reserve and the possibility of repeat operations. Using sTAE as the main treatment against HCC, survival rates of more than 70% at 3 years were achieved.

References

1. Kobayashi K, Sugimoto T, Makino H, Kumagai M, Unoura M, Tanaka N, Kato Y, Hattori N (1985) Screening methods for early detection of hepatocellular carcinoma. Hepatology 5:1100–1105
2. Unoura M, Kaneko S, Matsushita E, Shimoda A, Takeuchi M, Adachi H, Kawai H, Urabe T, Yanagi M, Matsui O (1993) High-risk groups and screening strategies for early detection of hepatocellular carcinoma in patients with chronic liver disease. Hepatogastroenterology 40:305–310
3. Allison DJ, Jordan H, Hennessy O (1985) Therapeutic embolisation of the hepatic artery: a review of 75 procedures. Lancet 1:595–599
4. Chuang VP, Wallace S (1981) Hepatic artery embolization in the treatment of hepatic neoplasms. Radiology 140:51–58

5. Vetter D, Wenger JJ, Bergier JM, Doffoel M, Bockel R (1991) Transcatheter oily chemoembolization in the management of advanced hepatocellular carcinoma in cirrhosis: results of a Western comparative study in 60 patients. Hepatology 13:427–433

6. Wheeler PG, Melia W, Dubbins P, Jones B, Nunnerley H, Johnson P, Williams R (1979) Non-operative arterial embolisation in primary liver tumours. Br Med J 2:242–244

7. Yamada R, Sato M, Kawabata M, Nakatsuka H, Nakamura K, Takashima S (1983) Hepatic artery embolization in 120 patients with unresectable hepatoma. Radiology 148:397–401

8. Groupe d'Etude et de Traitement du Carcinome Hepatocellulaire (1995) A comparison of lipiodol chemoembolization and conservative treatment for unresectable hepatocellular carcinoma. N Engl J Med 332:1256–1261

9. Bronowicki JP, Vetter D, Dumas F, Boudjema K, Bader R, Weiss AM, Wenger JJ, Boissel P, Bigard MA, Doffoel M (1994) Transcatheter oily chemoembolization for hepatocellular carcinoma. A 4-year study of 127 French patients. Cancer 74:16–24

10. Kasugai H, Kojima J, Tatsuta M, Okuda S, Sasaki Y, Imaoka S, Fujita M, Ishiguro S (1989) Treatment of hepatocellular carcinoma by transcatheter arterial embolization combined with intraarterial infusion of a mixture of cisplatin and ethiodized oil. Gastroenterology 97:965–971

11. Liu CL, Fan ST (1997) Nonresectional therapies for hepatocellular carcinoma. Am J Surg 173:358–365

12. Nakamura H, Hashimoto T, Oi H, Sawada S (1989) Transcatheter oily chemoembolization of hepatocellular carcinoma. Radiology 170:783–786

13. Pelletier G, Roche A, Ink O, Anciaux ML, Derhy S, Rougier P, Lenoir C, Attali P, Etienne JP (1990) A randomized trial of hepatic arterial chemoembolization in patients with unresectable hepatocellular carcinoma. J Hepatol 11:181–184

14. Matsui O, Kadoya M, Yoshikawa J, Gabata T, Arai K, Demachi H, Miyayama S, Takashima T, Unoura M, Kogayashi K (1993) Small hepatocellular carcinoma: treatment with subsegmental transcatheter arterial embolization. Radiology 188:79–83

15. Kan Z, Ivancev K, Hagerstrand I, Chuang VP, Lunderquist A (1989) In vivo microscopy of the liver after injection of Lipiodol into the hepatic artery and portal vein in the rat. Acta Radiol 30:419–425

16. Nakamura H, Hashimoto T, Oi H, Sawada S (1988) Iodized oil in the portal vein after arterial embolization. Radiology 167:415–417

17. Nakamura H, Hashimoto T, Oi H, Sawada S, Furui S, Mizumoto S, Monden M (1990) Treatment of hepatocellular carcinoma by segmental hepatic artery injection of adriamycin-in-oil emulsion with overflow to segmental portal veins. Acta Radiol 31: 347–349

18. Murakami R, Yoshimatsu S, Yamashita Y, Sagara K, Arakawa A, Takahashi M (1994) Transcatheter hepatic subsegmental arterial chemoembolization therapy using iodized oil for small hepatocellular carcinomas. Correlation between lipiodol accumulation pattern and local recurrence. Acta Radiol 35:576–580

Clinical Significance of Liposome-Encapsulated OK-432 Injection with Simultaneous Interventional Radiological Treatment of Hepatocellular Carcinoma Based on Experimental Analysis of Liver-Associated Lymphocytes

Takafumi Ichida[1], Satoshi Yamagiwa[1], Kazunari Sato[1], Satoshi Sugahara[1], Kazuhiro Uehara[1], Tohru Ishikawa[1], Masashi Katoh[2], Hiroshi Satoh[2], and Hitoshi Asakura[1]

Summary. OK-432 is a biological response modifier used in Japan to augment host immunity and is known to increase the host antitumor response. Using liposomes, which are vesicles made of phospholipids that have a structure resembling the cell membrane, we encapsulated OK-432. Encapsulated OK-432 was injected into the tail veins of mice, and its effect was compared with that of unencapsulated OK-432 given intravenously. In mice receiving either form of OK-432, both natural killer (NK) and intermediate TCR cells (intrahepatic T cells generated by extrathymic differentiation) increased markedly in the liver, with the peak level occurring 3 days after administration. Both forms of OK-432 also increased cytotoxic activity against Yac-1 cells. The increase of cells and cytotoxic activity in the liver persisted for longer in mice receiving encapsulated OK-432 than in animals receiving unencapsulated OK-432. Because both NK and intermediate TCR cells play an important role in tumor immunity, it may be useful for the treatment of tumors, particularly hepatocellular carcinoma. Local recurrence rate of hepatocellular carcinoma treated with liposome-encapsulated OK-432 and simultaneous segmental lipiodol transcatheter arterial embolization (TAE) therapy was significantly lower than without OK-432 ($P < .02$).

Key words. OK-432 Liposome, Liver-associated lymphocytes, hepatocellular carcinoma, interventional radiology.

Introduction

OK-432 is a biological response modifier derived from the weakly virulent Su strain of *Streptococcus pyogenes*. It produces pronounced augmentation of host immunity and is known to have an antitumor effect [1–4]. OK-432 has shown a clear antitumor effect in clinical studies. Although it has been widely used in Japan as adjuvant chemotherapy for several cancers [5–9], it has not been as effective clinically as expected from the results of animal studies and side-effects prevent prolonged administration.

---

[1] Third Department of Internal Medicine and [2] Department of Pharmacy, Niigata University School of Medicine, 1-757 Asahimachi-Dori, Niigata 951-8510, Japan

Recent progress in drug delivery systems has made it possible to minimize side-effects and prolong the duration of action of various drugs. Liposomes are vesicles made of phospholipids with a structure that resembles the cell membrane [10]. To lessen side-effects and prolong the duration of action, liposomes containing OK-432 were prepared and evaluated in mice in the present study.

After satisfactory experimental results in mice, we set up a clinical trial to treat hepatocellular carcinoma with liposome-encapsulated OK-432. This clinical trial had the full approval of the institute committee for research of human subjects in our university.

Materials and Methods

Mice

C3H/HeN mice were used at the age of 5 to 12 weeks. All mice were housed under specific pathogen-free (SPF) conditions in the animal facility of Niigata University after being purchased from Clea Japan (Tokyo, Japan).

OK-432

OK-432, a penicillin- and heat-treated lyophilized preparation of the Su strain of *Streptococcus* group A3, was provided by Chugai Pharmaceutical Company (Tokyo, Japan). One Klinische Einheit unit (KE) corresponds to 0.1 mg of dried bacteria. The lyophilized preparation was suspended at a concentration of 1 KE per 0.2 ml of saline. Mice were injected intravenously through the tail vein at a dose of 1 KE per animal.

Liposome-Encapsulated OK-432

OK-432 (2 KE) was suspended in 2 ml of saline and was added to the ether solution. Then a liposome suspension was extruded from a special apparatus with a polycarbonate membrane (pore size: 100 nm) to form a monolayer liposome. Liposome-encapsulated OK-432 (OK-Lipo) formed by the process had a particle size of about 100–300 nm.

Experimental Schedule

OK-432 and OK-Lipo were administered intravenously to mice at a dose of 1 KE per animal on day 0. Mice were killed after 6h, 12h, 1 day, 3 days, 5 days, and 7 days. Mononuclear cells (MNC) were prepared from various organs and analyzed by flow cytometry and by a ^{51}Cr-release assay. Each group consisted of 3–5 mice and the experimental protocol was done three times.

Cell Preparations

The liver was pressed through a 200-gauge stainless steel mesh and then suspended in Eagle's MEM supplemented with 5mM HEPES (Nissui Pharmaceutical, Tokyo, Japan) and 2% heat-inactivated newborn calf serum. After washing, the cells were fractionated by centrifugation for 15min at 2000rpm [11].

Immunofluorescence Analysis

The surface phenotype of cells was determined using monoclonal antibodies with two-color or three-color immunofluorescence analysis [11]. The monoclonal antibodies used included fluorescein isothiocyanate (FITC)-, phycoerythrin (PE)-, or biotin-conjugated anti-CD3; anti-IL-2 receptor (β-chain); anti-B220; anti-TCR$\alpha\beta$; anti-TCR$\gamma\delta$; anti-CD4; and anti-CD8 (PharMingen, San Diego, CA, USA). Biotin-conjugated reagents were developed with PE-conjugated streptavidin (Becton-Dickinson, Mountain View, CA, USA). To prevent nonspecific binding, CD32/16 (2.4G2) was added before staining with the labeled mAbs. Fluorescence-positive cells were analyzed with a FACScan using Lysis II software (Becton-Dickinson).

^{51}Cr-Release Assay

Cytotoxicity was examined by a ^{51}Cr-release assay [12]. Fresh MNC were prepared from the liver and spleen as described above. ^{51}Cr-labeled YAC-1 cells (1×10^4/well) were incubated with effector cells at the indicated target-to-effector ratios for 4h at 37°C. After incubation, the radioactivity released into the supernatant was measured and the percent specific lysis was calculated.

Clinical Trials for the Treatment of Hepatocellular Carcinoma Utilizing Liposome-Encapsulated OK-432

Twenty-four hepatocellular carcinomas were enrolled in this trial. Group I patients received liposome-encapsulated OK-432 and segmental lipiodol TAE therapy simultaneously and group II patients received segmental lipiodol transarterial embolization (TAE) alone.

After treatment for 30 months, the local recurrence rate was studied by total imaging methods and tumor markers. Patient details are shown in Table 1. All patients had hepatocellular carcinoma associated with liver cirrhosis type C with Child status A.

Statistical Analysis

Statistical analysis was performed by Student's t-test and $P < .05$ was taken to indicate significance. The log rank test was used for statistical analysis of clinical data.

Table 1. Background of patients with hepatocellular carcinoma enrolling in this clinical trial

Group I: Hepatocellular carcinoma patients treated with liposome-encapsulated OK-432 and simultaneous segmental lipiodol TAE therapy

Clinical stage	Age	Sex	Recurrence	Follow-up period (months)	Background
I	76	M	(−)	18	LC(C)
	68	F	(−)	12	LC(C)
II	54	M	(+)	12	LC(C)
	75	M	(−)	10	LC(C)
	73	M	(+)	8	LC(C)
	49	M	(−)	12	LC(C)
	56	F	(+)	14	LC(C)
	62	M	(−)	18	LC(C)
	68	M	(−)	8	LC(C)
III	69	M	(+)	15	LC(C)
	72	M	(+)	26	LC(C)
	70	M	(+)	26	LC(C)

Group II: Hepatocellular carcinoma patients treated with segmental lipiodol TAE therapy without liposome-encapsulated OK-432

Clinical stage	Age	Sex	Recurrence	Follow-up period (months)	Background
I	53	M	(+)	20	LC(C)
	57	M	(+)	6	LC(C)
	60	F	(+)	8	LC(C)
II	67	F	(+)	53	LC(C)
	64	F	(+)	17	LC(C)
	62	M	(+)	18	LC(C)
	65	M	(+)	14	LC(C)
	75	M	(+)	12	LC(C)
	71	M	(+)	8	LC(C)
III	62	F	(+)	18	LC(C)
	65	M	(+)	3	LC(C)
	55	F	(+)	11	LC(C)

LC(C), liver cirrhosis type C.

Results

Identification of Natural Killer and Intermediate TCR Cells

Two-color staining of cells for CD3 and IL-2 receptor β-chain (IL-2Rβ) allowed natural killer (NK) cells to be distinguished as CD3⁻IL-2Rβ⁺ cells and conventional T cells as CD3⁺IL-2Rβ⁻ cells. The fraction marked with an arrowhead in Fig. 1 comprised T cells expressing CD3 at a somewhat lower level than conventional T cells or an intermedi-

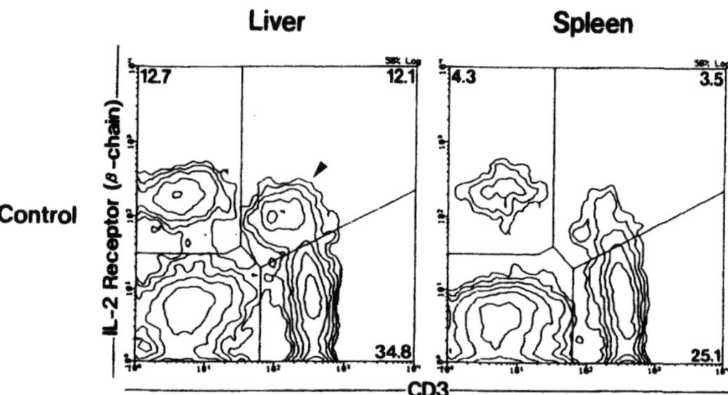

Fig. 1. Identification of natural killer cells and intermediate TCR cells in the livers and spleens of control mice. C3H/HeN mice aged 8 weeks were used. Mononuclear cells were prepared from the harvested livers and spleens. Two-color staining for CD3 and the IL-2 receptor β chain (IL-2Rβ) was performed. Numbers indicate the percentages of fluorescence-positive cells in the corresponding areas. Intermediate TCR cells (*arrowhead*) with intermediate levels of CD3 expression and constitutive IL-2Rβ expression was demonstrated to exist in the liver and was of extrathymic origin

ate level, even when expressing IL-2Rβ. When IL-2R is expressed in association with T cell activation, both IL-2Rα and IL-2Rβ are expressed concomitantly. Cells of this type were abundant in the liver. They are called intermediate TCR cells, and have been reported to be intrahepatic T cells that undergo extrathymic differentiation [13].

Phenotypic Analysis of MNC in Mice Liver after Intravenous Injection of Liposome-Encapsulated OK-432, Unencapsulated OK-432, and Empty Liposomes

In animals receiving unencapsulated OK-432, OK-Lipo, and empty liposomes, NK and intermediate TCR cells were counted in the liver at intervals after injection (Table 2). In animals receiving unencapsulated OK-432, NK and intermediate TCR cells increased until 3 days after injection, and then decreased rapidly. At 5 and 7 days after injection, their levels were below those before injection. In animals receiving OK-Lipo, cells also increased until 3 days after injection. Although the peak level was approximately the same as in animals receiving unencapsulated OK-432, the subsequent decrease was slower. Seven days after injection of OK-Lipo, the cell levels were higher than before injection. Injection of empty liposomes increased the cell levels to some extent, and both NK and intermediate TCR cells remained elevated longer than after unencapsulated OK-432.

Augmentation of NK Activity in the Liver after Intravenous Injection of Liposome-Encapsulated OK-432 and Unencapsulated OK-432

Yac-1, as an NK-sensitive cell line, was used to assess cytotoxic activity following intravenous injection of OK-Lipo and unencapsulated OK-432. The cytotoxic activity in

Table 2. Phenotypic analysis of liver associated lymphocytes of mice after intravenous injection of liposome encapsulated OK-432, OK-432 alone and liposome

Time	Treatment	Positive and negative cells (%)		
		NK	Int TCR	High TCR
Day 0	Control	16.8 ± 8.0	10.9 ± 5.9	25.7 ± 4.9
Day 3	OK432	34.4 ± 6.8	14.0 ± 3.6	21.9 ± 5.3
	OK-Lipo	37.0 ± 1.5	15.4 ± 5.4	27.2 ± 3.0
	Lipo alone	27.5 ± 3.0	8.8 ± 1.1	18.9 ± 4.9
Day 5	OK432	18.4 ± 3.0	9.9 ± 0.3	24.6 ± 1.8
	OK-Lipo	25.3 ± 2.8	13.3 ± 2.0	27.5 ± 4.0
	Lipo alone	20.6 ± 1.3	10.7 ± 4.9	26.0 ± 4.6
Day 7	OK432	16.4 ± 2.7*	11.2 ± 4.2	30.0 ± 1.6
	OK-Lipo	21.8 ± 5.5*	12.3 ± 1.9	33.3 ± 6.9
	Lipo alone	18.6 ± 6.6	14.7 ± 8.3	24.1 ± 4.0

Data are the mean ± SD of 3–5 experiments.
OK-Lipo, liposome-encapsulated OK-432; Lipo alone, liposomes alone; NK, natural killer.
*$P < .01$.

the liver was $\geqq 90\%$ at 3 days after injection along with the increase of NK and intermediate TCR cells. Cytotoxic activity tended to decrease subsequently. The decrease after OK-Lipo was slower than that after unencapsulated OK-432. Seven days after injection, cytotoxic activity was significantly higher in the OK-Lipo group than in the unencapsulated OK-432 group ($P < .01$).

Clinical Results after Treatment with Liposome-Encapsulated OK-432

After treatment of patients with hepatocellular carcinoma using OK-Lipo and simultaneous segmented lipiodol TAE therapy or segmented lipiodol TAE therapy alone, periodical examination of tumor recurrence by ultrasound, CT scan, MRI, and tumor markers such as AFP and PIVKA II was performed. Local recurrence rates were significantly different between the two groups. Low local recurrence was observed in the Group I (log rank $P = .02$) (Figure 2).

Discussion

OK-432 is a biological response modifier commonly used in Japan. OK-432 is known to activate macrophages, NK cells, and LAK cells, and also induces the production of a variety of cytokines. In mice, intravenous injection of OK-432 has been reported to increase the number and cytotoxic activity of LAK cells in the spleen. In the present study, intravenous injection of OK-432 caused the numbers of NK and intermediate TCR cells to increase in the liver. Although OK-432 was administered systemically, it specifically increased NK and intermediate TCR cells in the liver. This specific effect

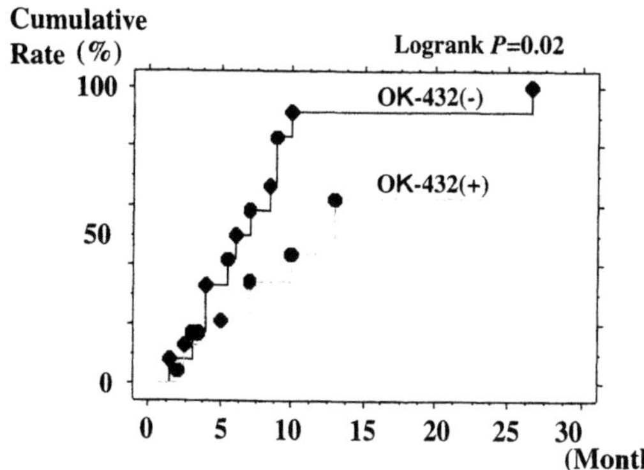

Fig. 2. Local recurrence rates in patients with hepatocellular carcinoma treated with liposome-encapsulated OK-432 and simultaneous segmented lipiodol TAE therapy or segmented lipiodol TAE therapy alone. A marked decrease in local recurrence rates was observed in the encapsulated OK-432 group

was only transient, therefore, OK-432 should be administered repeatedly or via a slow-release delivery system.

Liposomes have several advantages as a drug delivery system: they entrap both water- and lipid-soluble drugs easily without chemical modification, and encapsulation of drugs lessens their toxicity for normal tissues and prevents inactivation in the blood circulation [10]. In addition, most of the liposomes administered are rapidly entrapped by reticuloendothelial macrophages in the liver and spleen [14]. We prepared OK-Lipo to augment the action of OK-432 on the liver. When OK-Lipo was injected intravenously, the numbers of NK and intermediate TCR cells increased, particularly in the liver, but the subsequent decrease was slower with encapsulated OK-432. Thus, it was recognized that encapsulation prolonged the duration of action of OK-432. This extension of the duration of action was probably because phagocytosis of the liposomes by macrophages is necessary for activation of encapsulated OK-432, so sustained release of OK-432 may occur as a result of the gradual progression of phagocytosis.

Both NK and intermediate TCR cells have been reported to play an important role in tumor immunity. It was recently shown that these cells have undergone extrathymic differentiation in the liver [13,15], and they are known to have antitumor activity, particularly against tumor metastasis [16]. In the present study, OK-432 also increased numbers of intermediate TCR cells, although the effect was weaker than that on NK cells, suggesting that intermediate TCR cells play a role in the antitumor action of OK-432 in the liver. Cytotoxic activity increased in conjunction with the increase of NK and intermediate TCR cells after administration of unencapsulated OK-432 and OK-Lipo, and the increased cytotoxic activity was significantly more persistent when OK-Lipo was administered. Such increased cytotoxic activity may be related to an antitumor effect in the liver.

Use of OK-432 in the treatment of liver tumors, particularly hepatocellular carcinoma, has been reported by many researchers [17]. Various problems with OK-432 have been mentioned. For example, it causes side-effects such as fever and has no direct cytocidal action. In some studies, OK-432 did not improve the overall outcome [18]. Kanai et al. reported that transarterial immunoembolization with OK-432 and fibrinogen was effective, but caused fever in 100% of the patients treated [19]. If OK-Lipo is used in place of unencapsulated OK-432, systemic side effects such as fever will be lessened because there is little extravasation of the drug. In the present study, liposome-encapusulated OK-432 administration did not caused severe side-effects and led to a low rate of local recurrence.

OK-Lipo has advantages over conventional OK-432 because in addition to a liver-specific increase in the number and cytotoxic activity of NK and intermediate TCR cells, its effects are more persistent and it causes fewer systemic side-effects than conventional OK-432. Therefore, OK-Lipo is likely to be useful in the treatment of liver tumors.

References

1. Bonavida B, Katz J, Hoshino T (1986) Mechanism of NK activation by OK-432 (*Streptococcus pyogenes*). Spontaneous release of NKCF and augmentation of NKCF production following stimulation with NK target cells. Cell Immunol 102:126–135
2. Saito M, Ichimura O, Kataoka M, Kataoka M, Moriya Y, Ueno K, Sugawara Y, Nanjo M, Ishida N (1986) Pronounced antitumor effect of LAK-like cells induced in the peritoneal cavity of mice after intraperitoneal injection of OK-432, a killed streptococcal preparation. Cancer Immunol Immunother 22:161–168
3. Shimoda K, Saito T, Kobayashi M, Nomoto K (1992) Effective in vivo induction of lymphokine-activated killer (LAK) cells by pretreatment with a streptococcal preparation, OK-432. Biotherapy 5:63–69
4. Wakasugi H, Kasahara T, Minato N, Hamuro J, Miyata M, Morioka Y (1982) In vitro potentiation of human natural killer cell activity by a streptococcal preparation, OK-432: interferon and interleukin-2 participation in the stimulation with OK-432. J Natl Cancer Inst 69:807–815
5. Watanabe Y, Iwa T (1984) Clinical value of immunotherapy for lung cancer by streptococcal preparation OK-432. Cancer 53:248–253
6. Mukai M, Kubota S, Morita S, Akanuma A (1995) A pilot study of combination therapy of radiation and local administration of OK-432 for esophageal cancer. Cancer 75:2276–2280
7. Tanaka N, Gouchi A, Ohara T, Mannami T, Konaga E, Fuchimoto S, Sato K, Orita K (1994) Intratumoral injection of a streptococcal preparation , OK-432, before surgery for gastric cancer. Cancer 74:3097–3103
8. Fujita K (1987) The role of adjunctive immunotherapy in superficial bladder cancer. Cancer 59:2027–2030
9. Maehara Y, Okuyama T, Kakeji Y, Baba H, Furusawa M, Sugimachi K (1994) Postoperative immunochemotherapy including streptococcal lysate OK-432 is effective for patients with gastric cancer and serosal invasion. Am J Surg 168:36–40
10. Baugham AD, Standish M, Watkins JC (1995) Diffusion of univalent ions across the lamelae of swollen phospholipid. J Mol Biol 13:238–252
11. Watanabe H, Miyaji C, Kawachi Y, Iiai T, Ohtsuka K, Iwanaga T, Takahashi-Iwanaga T, Abo T (1995) Relationships between intermediate TCR cells and NK1.1$^+$ T cells in various immune organs. NK1.1$^+$ T cells are present within a population of intermediate TCR cells. J Immunol 155:2972–2983
12. Moroda T, Iiai T, Kawachi Y, Kawamura T, Hatakeyama K, Abo T (1996) Restricted appearance of self-reactive clones into intermediate T cell receptor cells in neonatally thymectomized mice with autoimmune disease. Eur J Immunol 26:3084–3091
13. Sato K, Ohtsuka K, Hasegawa K, Yamagiwa S, Watanabe H, Abo T (1995) Evidence for extrathymic generation of intermediate T cell receptor cells in the liver revealed in

thymectomized, irradiated mice subjected to bone marrow transplantation. J Exp Med 182:759–767
14. Segal AW, Wills EJ, Richmond JE, Slavin G, Black CD, Gregoriadis G (1974) Morphological observations on the cellular and subcellular destination of intravenously administered liposomes. Br J Exp Path 55:320–327
15. Watanabe H, Miyaji C, Seki S, Abo T (1996) C-kit[+] stem cells and thymocyte precursors in the liver of adult mice. J Exp Med 184:687–693
16. Takeda K, Seki S, Ogasawara K, Anzai R, Hashimoto W, Sugiura K, Takahashi M, Saitoh M, Kumagai K (1996) Liver NK1.1[+]CD4[+] cells activated by IL-12 as a major effector in inhibition of experimental tumor metastasis. J Immunol 156:3366–3373
17. Imaoka S, Sasaki Y, Matsui Y (1982) Evaluation of intratumoral injection of an immunopotentiator (OK-432) in patients with hepatocellular carcinoma. J Jpn Soc Cancer Therapy 17:1957–1963
18. Suto T, Fukuda S, Moriya N, Moriya N, Watanabe Y, Sasaki D, Yoshida Y, Sakata Y (1994) Clinical study of biological response modifier as maintenance therapy for hepatocellular carcinoma. Cancer Chemother Pharmacol 33(Suppl.):S145–148
19. Kanai T, Monden M, Sakon M, Gotoh M, Umeshita K, Hasuike Y, Nakano H, Monden T, Murakami T, Nakamura H (1994) New development of transarterial immunoembolization (TIE) for therapy of hepatocellular carcinoma with intrahepatic metastases. Cancer Chemother Pharmacol 33(Suppl.):S48–54

Phase II Trial of Hepatic Arterial Infusion Chemotherapy Using Cisplatin and 5-Fluorouracil in Patients with Advanced Hepatocellular Carcinoma

Masatoshi Tanaka, Eiji Ando, Sigeru Yutani, Kazuta Fukumori, Ryoko Kuromatsu, Yoshihiro Shimauchi, Hiroaki Nagamatsu, Satoshi Matsugaki, Satoshi Itano, Naohumi Ono, Shyotaroh Sakisaka, and Michio Sata

Summary. We investigated the effect of hepatic artery infusion (HAI) chemotherapy on advanced hepatocellular carcinoma. Ten milligrams per hour of cisplatin for 1 h and subsequently 250 mg/h for 5 h of 5-fluorouracil were administered using a subcutaneously implanted vascular access device (an injection port) for 5 consecutive days followed by 2 days rest. One course consisted of repetition of the above dosage regimen for 4 weeks. We treated 77 patients with advanced hepatocellular carcinoma (HCC), excluding nodular-type tumors indicated for chemoembolization, percutaneous ethanol injection therapy, or hepatic resection. Vascular invasion was seen in 28 patients and distant metastasis was seen in 7 patients. Of patients with advanced HCC, 77% were at tumor stage IV. Ten patients (13%) had a complete response, 25 (32%) had a partial response, 30 (39%) exhibited no change, and 12 (16%) had progressive disease. The response rate was thus 46%. Estimated 1-year, 2-year, and 3-year survival by the Kaplan-Meier method in 77 patients was 56%, 28%, and 19%, respectively. According to a multivariate analysis, the effects of initial therapy ($P < .0001$) and the Child-Pugh grade ($P = .0012$) were significant prognostic factors. A survival benefit was noted in patients with portal vein invasion (1-year survival rate: 43%, 2-year survival rate: 24%) when compared with reported results, and HAI was considered to be the first choice for unresectable cases. Adverse reactions of patients were tolerable and included transient nausea, loss of appetite, and mild thrombocytopenia. In conclusion, HAI chemotherapy with the regimen described achieved favorable results, and is useful in treating patients with advanced HCC not indicating chemoembolization, hepatic resection, or ethanol injection therapy.

Key words. Hepatocellular carcinoma, Hepatic arterial infusion chemotherapy, cisplatin, 5-Fluorouracil

Introduction

Advanced hepatocellular carcinoma associated with vascular invasion and/or multiple hepatic metastasis is often accompanied by distant metastasis. However, the cause of death in most patients is still cancer associated with progressive hepatic lesions or

Second Department of Medicine, Kurume University School of Medicine, Kurume 830-0011, Japan

liver failure [1]. Hence, improved therapy for such hepatic lesions is required to increase patient survival. We investigated the effects of hepatic arterial infusion (HAI) chemotherapy on advanced hepatocellular carcinoma (HCC). To potentiate the anti-cancer effect of the drugs and to relieve side effects on the basis of biochemical modulation, an intermittent and frequent low-dose chemotherapy regimen using cisplatin and 5-fluorouracil (5-FU) was performed [2,3]. Drugs were administered using a subcutaneously implanted vascular access device (an injection port) [4].

Patients and Methods

HAI chemotherapy was performed on 77 patients with advanced HCC excluding nodular-type tumors indicated for hepatic artery embolization. The background and tumor factors of the 77 patients treated are shown in Table 1. Portal vein tumor thrombus was seen in 28 patients and distant metastasis was seen in 7 patients. Of patients with advanced HCC, 77% were at tumor stage IV. The deadline for entry was December 31, 1996 and the final day of follow up was December 31, 1997. Therapeutic effect was judged at its maximum 3–6 months after completion of therapy by imaging diagnosis on the basis of efficacy criteria by the Liver Cancer Study Group of Japan.

The drug protocol consisted of the daily administration of cisplatin (10 mg/h for 1 h on days 1 to 5) and the subsequent infusion of 5-FU (50 mg/h for 5 h on days 1 to 5). Days 6 and 7 were rest days. This course was repeated for 4 weeks based on patient performance status, hepatic function, and adverse reactions. Additional therapy after initial HAI chemotherapy was performed according to the following principles: (1) Maintenance therapy was not performed in complete-response patients, and the same therapy was repeated if recurrence was confirmed. (2) Maintenance therapy was not performed in partial-response patients or no-change patients. (3) Additional therapy such as hepatic resection, percutaneous ethanol injection therapy [5], or chemoembolization [6] was performed on partial-response patients if these therapies were

Table 1. Patient profiles and tumor factors

Patients	77	Gross classification		Portal vein invasion	
Age (mean)	64.6 ± 7.6	Nodular and single	8	Present/absent	28/49
Gender		Nodular and multiple	48	Distant metastasis	
Male/female	61/16	Massive, diffuse	21	Present/absent	7/70
Virus marker		Tumor stage			
HCVAb$^+$/	67/9	I/II/III/IV	0/2/16/59		
HBsAg$^+$		Tumor location	21/56		
Clinical stage		Uni-/bilobular			
CS1/CS2/CS3	19/47/11	Range			
Serum AFP level	Mean				
(ng/ml)	12 612		4–470 000		
Serum DCP level					
(AU/ml)	17.1		0.06–177		

deemed suitable to the patient's condition after initial therapy. If HAI chemotherapy was deemed suitable to the patients' condition, the same therapy was repeated after tumor recurrence was confirmed. (4) Drugs were immediately changed in patients with progressive disease.

Results

Effect of Initial Therapy and Patient Survival Rates

Ten patients had a complete response, 25 patients had a partial response, 30 patients had no change, and 12 patients had progressive disease. The response rate was thus 46%. Estimated 1-year, 2-year, and 3-year survival by the Kaplan-Meier method in 77 patients was 56%, 28%, and 19%, respectively.

Prognostic Factors

Prognostic factors were investigated by the Kaplan-Meier method and the results are shown in Table 2. These prognostic factors were tested by multivariate analysis with

Table 2. Factors relating cumulative survival of patients with HCC using univariate analysis (Kaplan–Meier method)

Factor	Survival (%)			
	1-year	2-year	3-year	*P*-value
Total cases (77)	55.8	27.6	18.3	
Treatment				*P* = .0012
Complete (61)	63.9	31.6	19.4	
Incomplete (16)	18.8	12.5	12.5	
Effect				*P* < .0001
CR (10)	90.0	90.0	78.8	
PR (25)	68.0	24.8	12.4	
NC (30)	56.7	23.3	8.0	
PD (12)	8.0	0.0	0.0	
Clinical stage				*P* = .0009
I (19)	89.5	57.9	39.1	
II (47)	48.9	23.0	16.1	
III (11)	36.4	0.0	0.0	
Tumor stage				*P* = .0089
II and III (18)	77.8	55.6	47.6	
IV (59)	50.8	21.1	12.3	
Distant metastasis				*P* = .004
Present (7)	28.6	0.0	0.0	
Absent (70)	60.0	32.1	21.9	
Portal thrombosis				*P* = .2231
Present (28)	42.9	23.6	19.6	
Absent (49)	65.3	32.4	19.9	

CR, complete response; PR, partial response; NC, no change; PD, progressive disease.

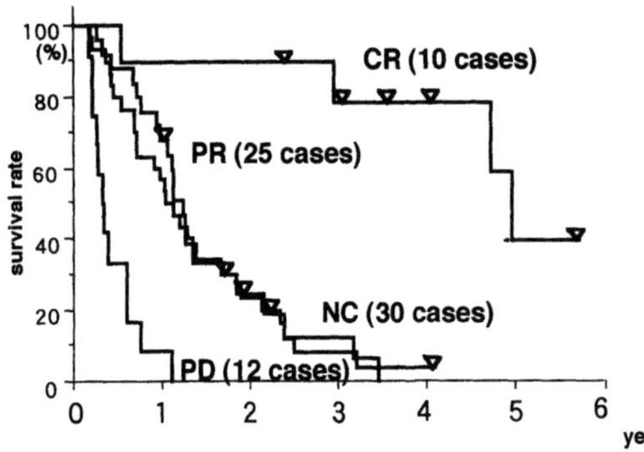

Fig. 1. Cumulative survival rate after hepatic arterial infusion chemotherapy using CDDP/5-FU for advanced HCC in relation to clinical effects

proportional hazard models. Effects of initial therapy ($P < .0001$) and clinical stage ($P = .0012$) were significant prognostic factors.

When prognosis was investigated by the presence of portal vein invasion, estimated 1-year and 2-year survival rates were 43% and 24%, respectively, and there was a difference by interval estimation in 1-year survival rates, but no significant difference in 2-year or 3-year survival rates. When compared with reported results [7,8], a survival benefit was noted in patients with portal vein invasion, and HAI chemotherapy using cisplatin and 5-FU was considered to be the first choice for unresectable cases.

As a result of analyzing survival rates in terms of the effect of initial therapy (Fig. 1), it was confirmed that patients with a complete response could be fully controlled by repeat treatment after detection of recurrence. There was no significant difference in survival rates between patients with a partial response and patients with no change, and it was revealed that some patients with a partial response were unresponsive to repeated HAI chemotherapy. It was considered that maintenance therapy was required for patients with a partial response.

Complications and Adverse Reactions

The complications and adverse reactions in 77 patients and 118 treatments were studied. As shown in Table 3, complications were caused mainly by technical problems associated with the indwelling of the catheter. The complication occurring most frequently was fever, probably caused by contamination of the catheter or an injection port. These infections were frequently found in patients at clinical stage III. The incidence of other complications, such as dislocation of the tip of the catheter or leakage at the connector, was low because of recent improvements in instruments and techniques relating to indwelling catheters.

As shown in Table 4, the most frequently occurring adverse reactions were early gastrointestinal symptoms, i.e., nausea, presumably caused by cisplatin; epigastric pain accompanying acute gastritis caused by arterial infusion of anticancer drugs, frequently occurring within 2 weeks of the start of arterial infusion; and anorexia, frequently occurring 2 weeks or more after the start of arterial infusion. Most side effects occurring at the later stage of the therapy can be overcome by thorough explanation to patients in advance, but in this study, the therapy had to be discontinued because of the development of hypoalbuminemia accompanying anorexia. Caution should be

Table 3. Summary of complications at initial treatment

Complications	Number (%) of patients
Infections	6 (7.7%)
Obstruction of devices	4 (5.2%)
Dislocation of catheter	2 (2.6%)
Leakage	6 (7.7%)
Total	11 (14%)

Table 4. Summary of adverse reactions on initial treatment

Adverse reactions	Grade (ECOG)				
	1	2	3	4	
Nausea	8	3			11
Appetite loss	12	11			23
Obstruction of hepatic artery				1	1[a]
Gastric ulcer	2				2
Duodenal ulcer	1	2			3
Stomatitis	2				2
Diarrhea		1			1
Leukopenia			2		2
Thrombocytopenia			3	1	4
Jaundice (>2.0 mg/ml)			1		1
Creatinine elevation (>2.0)	1				1
Total					34 (44%)

[a] In 7 cases, we experienced obstruction of hepatic artery with repeated hepatic arterial infusion.

exercised when any of the following occur: hemorrhagic gastric ulcer, marrow depression after the end of therapy, and especially thrombocytopenia. Increased blood creatinine may occur, although it occurred in only 1 of 77 patients in this study. When patients respond to the therapy, transfusion, administration of diuretic agents, and reduction of dose of cisplatin were performed in our department, but continuation of the therapy should be determine in consideration of the prognosis.

Vascular occlusion presumably caused by administration of anticancer drugs occurred in 7 patients though it occurred in only 1 patient at initial therapy. Vascular occlusion greatly disturbs continuation of the therapy. To reduce this side effect as much as possible, indwelling catheter techniques should be used that do not injure the vessel, e.g., the side hole method in which the catheter is fixed to the gastroduodenal artery or in which the catheter is inserted into the hepatic artery.

Sixteen patients could not achieve the dose of 200 mg of cisplatin and 5000 mg of 5-FU in one session (4 weeks) of initial therapy (21%). Five out of 11 patients at clinical stage III could not finish the protocol completely. Survival rates of stage-III patients overlapped, but this was probable because of the small number of patients. Because survival benefits were not noted in patients at clinical stage III, such patients will not receive the therapy in the future.

Discussion

Regional hepatic artery infusion is a reasonable drug delivery system for cancer limited to the liver because most advanced HCCs are nourished from arterial blood and so high hepatic drug concentrations can be maintained. In addition, if drugs are used with a high adsorption rate in the liver, systemic drug concentration is lower than with systemic administration, and the severity of side effects on other organs is reduced owing to the first-pass effect. As methods of administration of anticancer drugs, continuous artery infusion or frequent artery infusion using an injection port and chemolipiodolization [9] are often performed. The present study is a retrospective analysis of a phase II study using an intermittent and frequent low-dose HAI chemotherapy regime of cisplatin and 5-FU for advanced HCC.

From the present phase II study, a survival benefit was noted in patients with a complete response (disappearance of tumor staining in the liver by diagnostic imaging). It is important, as part of the overall strategy in patients with a partial response, to choose suitable additional therapy, such as hepatic resection, radiofrequency ablation, or chemoembolization, that may lead to a complete disappearance of tumor in the liver (complete response).

In patients with a partial response for whom there was no suitable additional therapy, there was no significant difference in survival between patients with a partial response and patients with no change. Maintenance therapy for patients with a partial response is important, and from 1996 we started chemo-lipiodolization therapy from an injection port as maintenance in patients with a partial response or no change. We have repeatedly performed chemolipiodolization with epirubicin or carboplatin and Lipiodol every 2 or 3 weeks in patients with a partial response or no change, according to their tumor stage. We are investigating the effect of maintenance therapy with a target total dose of 1500 mg of carboplatin and 200 mg of epirubicin. However, further follow up is required.

Survival benefits were also noted in advanced HCC with portal vein tumor thrombus, which is a significant prognostic factor of poor outcome [10]. According to our results, HAI chemotherapy using cisplatin and 5-FU is a first choice for advanced and unresectable HCCs with portal vein tumor thrombus. Finally, the HAI chemotherapy described here is not considered suitable for patients with HCC with poor liver function, such as patients at clinical stage III.

References

1. Okada S (1998) Chemotherapy in hepatocellular carcinoma. Hepato-Gastroenterlogy 45:1259–1263
2. Scanlon KJ, Newman EM, Lu Y, et al. (1986) Biochemical basis for cisplatin and 5-fluorouracil synergism in human ovarian cancer. Proc Natl Acad Sci USA 83:8923–8925
3. Shirasaka T, Shimamoto Y, Ohshima H, et al. (1993) Metabolic basis of the synergistic antitumor activities of 5-fluorouracil and cisplatin in rodent tumor model in vivo. Cancer Chemother Pharmacol 32:167–172

4. Ando E, Yamshita F, Tanaka M (1997) A novel chemotherapy for advanced hepatocellular carcinoma with tumor thrombosis of the main portal of the portal vein. Cancer 79:1890–1896
5. Ehara M, Ohto M, Sugiura N, et al. (1990) Percutaneous ethanol injection for the treatment of small hepatocellular carcinoma: study of 95 patients. J Gastroenterol Hepatol 5:616–626
6. Yamada R, Sato M, Kawabata M, et al. (1983) Hepatic artery embolization in 120 patients with unresectable hepatoma. Radiology 148:397–401
7. Okada S, Okazaki N, Nose N, et al. (1992) Prognostic factors in patients with hepatocellular carcinoma receiving systemic chemotherpy. Hepatology 16:112–117
8. Chen SC, Hsieh MY, Chuang WL, et al. (1994) Development of portal vein invasion and its outcome in hepatocellular carcinoma treated by transcatheter arterial chemoembolization. J Gastroentrol Hepatol 9:1–6
9. Konno T (1992) Targeting chemotherapy for hepatoma: arterial administration of anticancer drugs dissolved in Lipiodol. Eur J Cancer 28:403–409
10. Akashi Y, Koreeda C, Enomoto S, et al. (1991) Prognosis of unresectable hepatocellular carcinoma: an evaluation based on multivariate analysis of 90 cases. Hepatology 14:262–268

Surgical Treatment of Hepatocellular Carcinoma

MASAAKI OKA, MINEKATSU NISHIDA, and YOSHITAKA MAEDA

Summary. Hepatic resection is currently performed for the treatment of hepatocellular carcinoma (HCC), which is associated with a high incidence of postoperative recurrence. The aim of this study was to clarify the prognostic factors after hepatic resection for HCC. A total of 144 patients who underwent hepatic resection for HCC were studied. Eight factors including albumin, tumor size, intrahepatic metastasis (IM), invasion into the portal vein (Vp), type of hepatectomy, operative time, blood loss, and tumor margin were analyzed with multivariate analysis using a stepwise multivariate logistic regression model to evaluate the prognostic factors after hepatic resection. The relationship between operative procedures and the type of treatment modalities was also investigated, and the outcome of treatment modalities was analyzed using the survival rate after recurrence. Multivariate analysis revealed the type of hepatectomy, Vp, and IM to be independent factors related to recurrence and prognosis. The 5-year survival rate in patients without Vp and without IM was significantly higher than in patients with Vp and with IM ($P < .05$). The 5-year survival rate and 5-year disease-free survival rate in patients who underwent subsegmentectomy or segmentectomy or lobectomy (anatomic resection) was significantly higher than in patients who underwent partial resection ($P < .01$ and $P < .05$). Eleven (31.4%) patients with intrahepatic recurrence after anatomic resection were treated with repeat hepatectomy but only 2 (8.3%) after nonanatomic resection. Moreover, repeat hepatectomy was significantly related to the prognosis after recurrence compared with chemolipiodolization and locoregional chemotherapy ($P < .05$). These results suggest that anatomic resection, which was related to a low recurrence rate as well as a greater chance of reresection, may be a useful surgical treatment for hepatocellular carcinoma.

Key words. Hepatocellular carcinoma, Hepatectomy, Invasion into the portal vein, Intrahepatic metastasis, Survival rate

Department of Surgery II, Yamaguchi University School of Medicine, 1144 Kogushi, Ube, Yamaguchi 755-8505, Japan

Introduction

Hepatocellular carcinoma (HCC) is one of the most common fatal cancers in the world. Great progress has been made in its diagnosis and treatment, and the development of noninvasive diagnostic techniques such as ultrasonography (US), computed tomography (CT), and magnetic resonance imaging (MRI) have contributed to its earlier diagnosis, which has increased the number of resectable cases. Hepatectomy has been accepted as the means of cure for patients with HCC [1,2]. However, long-term results remain unsatisfactory. Intrahepatic recurrence following surgery is the main cause of poor prognosis for patients with resectable HCC [3], and the type of hepatectomy has little influence on recurrence or long-term survival [4,5]. It is therefore necessary to identify factors that can predict tumor recurrence and prognosis of patients.

Ng et al. [6] reported that tumor encapsulation and heavy intratumor inflammatory infiltration were independent favorable factors related to tumor recurrence and that negative resection margin and heavy intratumor inflammatory infiltration were independent favorable factors correlated with survival in patients who had undergone hepatectomy. El-Assal et al. [7] have demonstrated the usefulness of a scoring system using a variety of pathological factors for prediction of recurrence and disease-free survival after curative hepatectomy in HCC patients. In the current study, we investigated the clinicopathological factors affecting tumor recurrence and prognosis in 144 patients who underwent hepatic resection for HCCs using multivariate analysis.

Prognostic Factors After Hepatic Resection for HCC

Between June 1991 and April 1998, 144 patients with HCC who underwent hepatic resection at the Department of Surgery II, Yamaguchi University School of Medicine, were selected. Our criteria for performing hepatectomy in patients with chronic liver disease were as follows: ascites were absent or controllable, the serum total bilirubin level was less than 2.0 mg/dl, prothrombin time was more than 50%, and the plasma retention of indocyanine green 15 min after injection was less than 40%. The type of hepatectomy such as lobectomy, segmentectomy, subsegmentectomy, and partial resection was decided according to these four factors.

Subsegmentectomy and segmentectomy (anatomic resection) were defined as complete anatomic resection of the area fed by the portal branches [8,9]. The appropriate segment was identified as the discolored area that was obtained by occlusion of the segmental glissonean pedicle at the hilum. The subsegment was identified in the same manner by occlusion of the subsegmental glissonean pedicle, which was exposed at the peripheral side from the segmental glissonean pedicle. Liver transection was usually required to expose the subsegmental glissonean pedicle. Tumor included in the discolored area was confirmed using ultrasound. Liver transection was carried out by cautery with irrigation forceps (CIF) [10], which was developed in our department.

Basically, Pringle's maneuver was not applied for liver transection to avoid ischemic and reperfusion injury.

Multivariate Analysis

Univariate analysis using 17 factors including age, sex, viral type, associated liver diseases, albumin, bilirubin, platelet, alanine aminotransferase (ALT), ICG15R, alphafetoprotein, tumor size, invasion into the portal vein (Vp), intrahepatic metastasis (IM), type of hepatectomy, operative time, blood loss, and tumor margin was performed (data not shown). From these factors, eight variables such as albumin, tumor size, IM, Vp, type of hepatectomy, operative time, blood loss, and tumor margin were selected and analyzed with multivariate analysis using a stepwise multivariate logistic regression model to evaluate the prognostic factors after hepatic resection. Multivariate analysis revealed the type of hepatectomy, Vp, and IM to be independent factors related to recurrence and prognosis (Table 1). Multivariate analysis for prognostic factors after hepatectomy in HCC patients has been reported in various series (Table 2) [1,6,11–20]. From these reports, vascular invasion including Vp and IM, tumor size, and negative surgical margin may be independent factors. Only our data demonstrated the type of hepatectomy to be an independent factor.

Invasion into the Portal Vein

The 3-year and 5-year survival rate in patients without Vp (87.2% and 59.0%, respectively) was significantly higher than in patients with Vp (54.4% and 36.2%) ($P < .05$) (Fig. 1). The tendency to grow into the portal vein, hepatic vein, or biliary duct is a widely accepted pathological characteristic of HCC [21,22]. Vp occurs frequently at an early stage and leads to an early intrahepatic metastasis (IM) through the portal vein, which is the main draining route of HCC.

Intrahepatic Metastasis

The 3-year and 5-year survival rate in patients without IM (84.0% and 60.3%, respectively) was significantly higher than in patients with IM (58.0% and 34.9%, respectively) ($P < .05$) (Fig. 2).

Table 1. Independent factors related to survival using multivariate analysis

Variables	Coefficient	Relative risk	P value
Type of hepatectomy			
Anatomic	1.679	4.704	$P = .0009$
Partial			
Vp			
Positive	2.348	5.771	$P = .0001$
Negative			
IM			
Positive	1.440	3.321	$P = .0049$
Negative			

Vp, invasion into the portal vein; IM, intrahepatic metastasis.

Table 2. Multivariate analyses of independent factors related to recurrence and survival

Authors	Significant factors
Yamanaka et al. [11]	Vp, IM, tumor size, negative resection margin
Lai et al. [12]	Negative resection margin, encapsulation
Calvet et al. [13]	Bilirubin, ascites, toxic syndrome, blood urea nitrogen, tumor size, gamma-glutamyltranspeptidase, age, serum sodium, presence of metastases
Izumi et al. [14]	Vp
Chou et al. [15]	Negative hepatitis B surface antigen (HbsAg)
Vauthey et al. [16]	Vp
Ng et al. [6]	Encapsulation, heavy intratumor inflammatory infiltration, negative resection margin
Lee et al. [1]	Functional liver reserve, negative resection margin
Arii et al. [17]	Alpha-fetoprotein, tumor size, number of tumors, liver cirrhosis, age, surgical curability, Vp
Nonami et al. [18]	Tumor size, multiple gross tumors, negative resection margin, Child classification
Ikeda et al. [19]	Diabetes mellitus, intrahepatic metastasis
Anonymous [20]	Child–Pugh stage, tumor morphology, alpha-fetoprotein, Vp
Our results	IM, Vp, anatomic resection

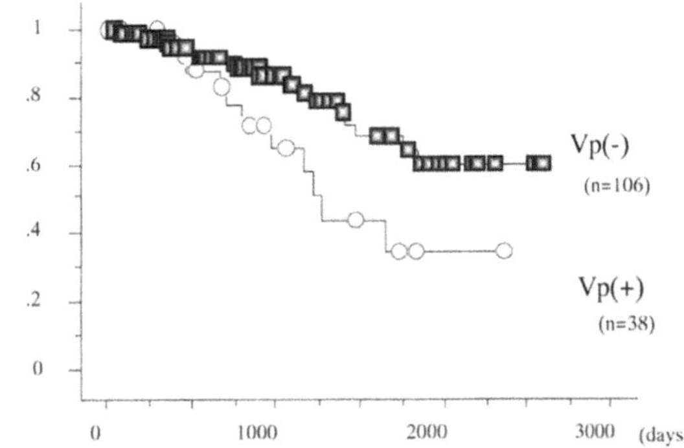

Fig. 1. Cumulative survival curve in patients with and without invasion into the portal vein (*Vp*). *Circles*, Vp positive; *squares*, Vp negative ($P < .05$)

The Type of Hepatectomy

The 3-year and 5-year survival rate in patients who underwent subsegmentectomy or segmentectomy or lobectomy (anatomic resection) (87.1% and 72.1%) was significantly higher than in patients who underwent partial resection (61.3% and 29.0%) ($P < .01$) (Fig. 3). The 3-year and 5-year disease-free survival rate in patients who underwent anatomic resection (49.1% and 36.2%, respectively) was significantly higher than in patients who underwent partial resection (25.3% and 0%, respectively) ($P < .05$) (Fig. 4).

The relationship between the type of hepatectomy and recurrence or prognosis is still controversial. It has been reported that the type of hepatectomy has little influence on recurrence or long-term survival [4,5]. Takayama et al. [23] have reported that the 3-year and 5-year survival rate in patients who underwent subsegmentectomy (70%

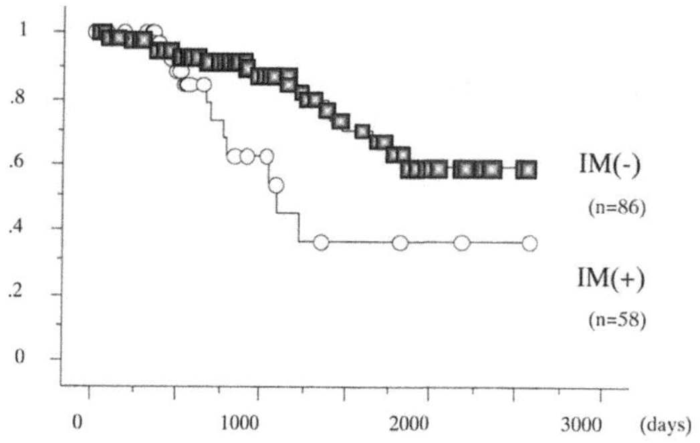

Fig. 2. Cumulative survival curve in patients with and without intrahepatic metastasis (*IM*). *Circles*, IM positive; *squares*, IM negative ($P < .05$)

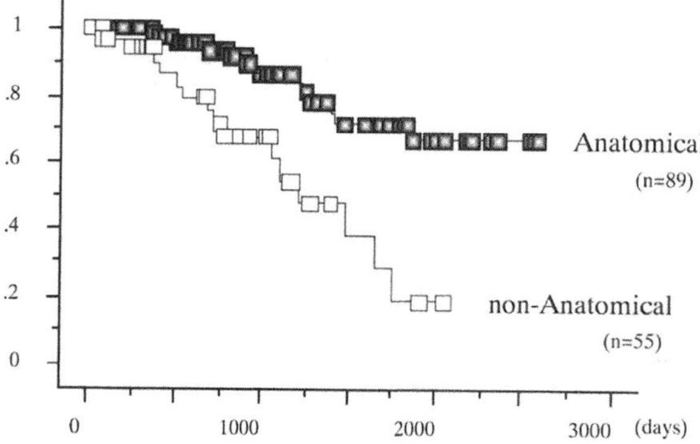

Fig. 3. Cumulative survival curve in patients who underwent anatomic resection (*closed squares*) and those who underwent nonanatomic resection (*open squares*) ($P < .01$)

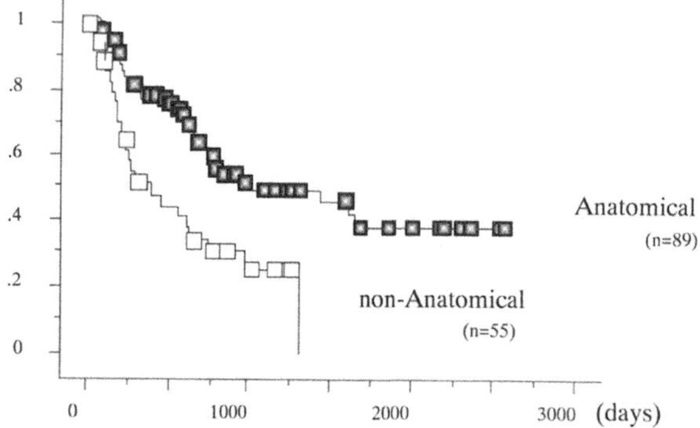

Fig. 4. Cumulative disease-free survival curve in patients who underwent anatomic resection (*closed squares*) and those who underwent nonanatomic resection (*open squares*) ($P < .05$)

and 51%, respectively) was significantly higher than in patients who underwent partial resection (64% and 38%, respectively). Miyagawa and Kawasaki [24] also have reported that the type of hepatectomy (limited vs. subsegmentectomy or segmentectomy) significantly affected the cumulative survival and disease-free survival rates. Portal venous invasion or intrahepatic metastasis is one of the most important predictive variables for recurrence [11,14,16,17,19]. Our data were consistent with these previous reports. Yamamoto et al. [25] demonstrated that more than half of all the observed intrahepatic recurrences were either in the same Healey segment or in the segment contiguous to the primary resected site in the ipsilateral lobe. They suggested intrahepatic spread of HCC in a segment-by-segment manner via the portal venous system. Considering the possibility of portal system-based spread, complete removal of the portal area containing the tumor might be more important for curative resection than nonanatomic resection. In fact, our multivariate analysis revealed anatomic resection to be an independent factor related to survival and disease-free survival. The present study is the first report of the efficacy of anatomic resection for HCC using multivariate analysis.

Treatment for Local Recurrence After Hepatic Resection

Of 88 patients with intrahepatic recurrence, therapeutic strategies for recurrence were investigated in 59 patients who underwent curative resection (Table 3). Thirty-five of 81 patients undergoing anatomic resection had intrahepatic recurrence. In these patients, chemolipiodolization were performed in 16, loco-regional chemotherapy in 4, percutaneous ethanol injection/microwave coagulation therapy (PEI/MCT) in 3, and reresection in 11 (31.4%). Twenty-four of 38 patients having nonanatomic resection had intrahepatic recurrence. In these patients, chemolipiodolization was performed in 12, loco-regional chemotherapy in 6, PEI/MCT in 1, and reresection in 2 (8.3%). The incidence of repeat hepatectomy in patients treated with anatomic resection was significantly higher than in patients treated with nonanatomic resection ($P < .05$). Figure 5 shows the survival rate in each therapy after recurrence. Repeat hepatectomy significantly improved the prognosis after recurrence compared with chemolipiodolization and locoregional chemotherapy ($P < .05$).

A repeat hepatectomy for recurrent HCC has been established as the most effective treatment modality, whenever it is possible [26,27]. The results of the present study were consistent with these reports. Furthermore, we demonstrated that patients who underwent anatomic resection had more chances of treatment by repeat hepatectomy. This finding may explain why the 5-year survival rate in patients treated with anatomic resection was higher than in patients treated with nonanatomic resection.

Table 3. Treatment of reccurent tumor after curative hepatic resection for hepatocellular carcinome (HCC)

Therapy	Anatomic resection	Partial resection
Chemolipiodolization	16	12
Locoregional chemotherapy	4	6
Percutaneous ethanol injection/microwave coagulation therapy (PEI/MCT)	3	1
Reresection	11 (31.4%)	2 (8.3%)
Unknown	1	3

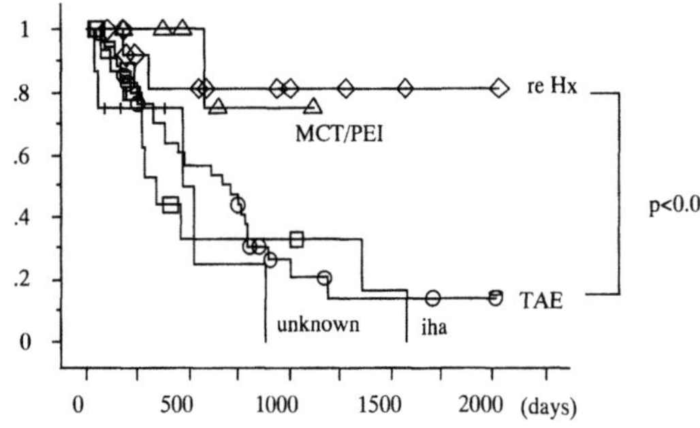

Fig. 5. Cumulative survival curve in each therapy for intrahepatic recurrence in patients who underwent hepatic resection. *re Hx*, repeat hepatic resection; *MCT*, microwave coagulation therapy; *PEI*, percutaneous ethanol injection; iha, loco-regional chemotherapy; *TAE*, chemolipiodolization

Conclusion

Because intrahepatic spread of hepatocellular carcinoma occurs in a segment-by-segment manner, anatomic hepatic resection should be selected within the hepatic functional reserve.

References

1. Lee NW, Wong J, Ong GB (1982) The surgical management of primary carcinoma of the liver. World J Surg 6:66–75
2. Okuda K, Ohtsuki T, Obata H, Tomimatsu M, Okazaki N, Hasegawa H, Nakajima Y, Ohnishi K (1985) Natural history of hepatocellular carcinoma and prognosis in relation to treatment. Study of 850 patients. Cancer (Phila) 56:918–928
3. Nagasue N, Uchida M, Makino Y, Takemoto Y, Yamanoi A, Hayashi T, Chang YC, Kohno H, Nakamura T, Yukaya H (1993) Incidence and factors associated with intrahepatic recurrence following resection of hepatocellular carcinoma. Gastroenterology 105:488–494
4. Harada T, Shigemura T, Kodama S, Higuchi T, Ikeda S, Okazaki M (1992) Hepatic resection is not enough for hepatocellular carcinoma. A follow-up study of 92 patients. J Clin Gastroenterol 14:245–250
5. Suenaga M, Nakao A, Harada A, Nonami T, Okada Y, Sugiura H, Uehara S, Takagi H (1992) Hepatic resection for hepatocellular carcinoma. World J Surg 16:97–104
6. Ng IO, Lai EC, Fan ST, Ng MM, So MK (1995) Prognostic significance of pathologic features of hepatocellular carcinoma. A multivariate analysis of 278 patients. Cancer (Phila) 76:2443–2448
7. El-Assal ON, Yamanoi A, Soda Y, Yamaguchi M, Yu L, Nagasue N (1997) Proposal of invasiveness score to predict recurrence and survival after curative hepatic resection for hepatocellular carcinoma. Surgery (St Louis) 122:571–577
8. Makuuchi M, Hasegawa H, Yamazaki S (1985) Ultrasonically guided subsegmentectomy. Surg Gynecol Obstet 161:346–350
9. Takasaki K (1998) Hepatic resection using glissonean pedicle transection. J Jpn Surg Soc 99:245–250
10. Takao T, Nishida M, Maeda Y, Oka M (1999) Effect of cautery with irrigation forceps in the rats. Eur Surg Res 31:173–179

11. Yamanaka N, Okamoto E, Toyosaka A, Mitunobu M, Fujihara S, Kato T, Fujimoto J, Oriyama T, Furukawa K, Kawamura E (1990) Prognostic factors after hepatectomy for hepatocellular carcinomas. A univariate and multivariate analysis. Cancer (Phila) 65:1104–1110

12. Lai EC, Ng IO, Ng MM, Lok AS, Tam PC, Fan ST, Choi TK, Wong J (1990) Long-term results of resection for large hepatocellular carcinoma: a multivariate analysis of clinicopathological features. Hepatology 11:815–818

13. Calvet X, Bruix J, Gines P, Bru C, Sole M, Vilana R, Rodes J (1990) Prognostic factors of hepatocellular carcinoma in the west: a multivariate analysis in 206 patients. Hepatology 12:753–760

14. Izumi R, Shimizu K, Ii T, Yagi M, Matsui O, Nonomura A, Miyazaki I (1994) Prognostic factors of hepatocellular carcinoma in patients undergoing hepatic resection. Gastroenterology 106:720–727

15. Chou FF, Sheen-Chen SM, Chen CL, Chen YS, Chen MJ (1994) Prognostic factors after hepatectomy for hepatocellular carcinoma. Hepato-Gastroenterology 41:419–423

16. Vauthey JN, Klimstra D, Franceschi D, Tao Y, Fortner J, Blumgart L, Brennan M (1995) Factors affecting long-term outcome after hepatic resection for hepatocellular carcinoma. Am J Surg 169:28–34

17. Arii S, Okamoto E, Imamura M (1996) Registries in Japan: current status of hepatocellular carcinoma in Japan. Liver Cancer Study Group of Japan. Semin Surg Oncol 12:204–211

18. Nonami T, Harada A, Kurokawa T, Nakao A, Takagi H (1997) Hepatic resection for hepatocellular carcinoma. Am J Surg 173:288–291

19. Ikeda Y, Shimada M, Hasegawa H, Gion T, Kajiyama K, Shirabe K, Yanaga K, Takenaka K, Sugimachi K (1998) Prognosis of hepatocellular carcinoma with diabetes mellitus after hepatic resection. Hepatology 27:1567–1571

20. Anonymous (1998) A new prognostic system for hepatocellular carcinoma: a retrospective study of 435 patients: the Cancer of the Liver Italian Program (CLIP) investigators. Hepatology 28:751–755

21. Nakashima T, Okuda K, Kojiro M, Jimi A, Yamaguchi R, Sakamoto K (1983) Pathology of hepatocellular carcinoma in Japan: 232 consecutive cases autopsied in ten years. Cancer (Phila) 51:863–877

22. Edmondson HA (1958) Tumors of the liver and intrahepatic bile ducts. Section VII, fasc 25. Armed Forces Institute of Pathology, Washington, DC, pp 32–109

23. Takayama T, Makuuchi M, Yamasaki S, Kosuge T, Yamamoto J, Shimada K (1998) Systematic resection for hepatocellular carcinoma. J Jpn Surg Soc 99:241–244

24. Miyagawa S, Kawasaki S (1998) Subsegmentectomy or segmentectomy in hepatocellular carcinoma. Hepato-Gastroenterology 45:2–6

25. Yamamoto J, Kosuge T, Takayama T, Shimada K, Yamasaki S, Ozaki H, Yamaguchi N, Makuuchi M (1996) Recurrence of hepatocellular carcinoma after surgery. Br J Surg 83:1219–1222

26. Suenaga M, Sugiura H, Kokuba Y, Uehara S, Kurumiya T (1994) Repeated hepatic resection for recurrent hepatocellular carcinoma in eighteen cases. Surgery (St Louis) 115:452–457

27. Shimada M, Takenaka K, Gion T, Fujiwara Y, Kajiyama K, Maeda T, Shirabe K, Nishizaki T, Yanaga K, Sugimachi K (1996) Prognosis of recurrent hepatocellular carcinoma: a 10-year surgical experience in Japan. Gastroenterology 111:720–726

Transjugular Intrahepatic Portosystemic Shunt for Patients with Hepatocellular Carcinoma

KENJI NAKAMURA, SUMIO TAKASHIMA, TOSHIO KAMINOU, YOUICHI KOHDA, MASAO HAMURO, SEISHO HAYASHI, ATSUKO MORIMOTO, RYOUICHI MATSUO, MICHIYO TANIGUCHI, and RYUSAKU YAMADA

Summary. Ten patients with hepatocellular carcinoma successfully underwent transjugular intrahepatic portosystemic shunt (TIPS) without technique-related complications. TIPS was indicated for massive ascites in six cases and ruptures of esophageal varices and hematemesis in four cases. Another two patients with massive ascites developed hepatocellular carcinoma between undergoing TIPS and follow-up observations after 12 and 30 months. In 10 of these 12 patients, the results of TIPS were satisfactory, having obtained good flow in the shunt and effective portal decompression. The gastrointestinal bleeding stopped in all four patients, and the uncontrollable ascites disappeared or decreased in six of the eight patients. Seven out of the 12 patients survived and were followed up for from 2 to 31 months after the TIPS procedure. After TIPS, five patients died due to tumor progression (three patients), hepatic failure (one patient) or acute hepatititis (one patient). In one other patient, the tumor ruptured one month after TIPS was performed. It is concluded that TIPS is a useful and safe treatment for portal hypertension, even in patients with hepatocellular carcinoma as long as it is not located in the puncture route. However, TIPS should be performed only in patients whose tumors have already been controlled by hepatic embolization and/or ethanol injection therapy. Careful follow-up observation is needed after the procedure on a long-term basis.

Key words. TIPS, Hepatocellular carcinoma, IVR, Portal hypertension

Introduction

In Japan, liver cirrhosis and portal hypertension due to hepatitis virus infection are frequently combined with hepatocellular carcinoma (HCC) [1–3]. Transcatheter arterial embolization (TAE) and percutaneous ethanol injection therapy (PEIT) are effective treatment for HCC and widely used not only in Japan but also in many other Asian countries. These techniques have prolonged the survival of patients

Department of Radiology, Osaka City University, 1-5-7 Asahimachi, Abeno-ku, Osaka 545-8585, Japan

with HCC [4–6]. However, patients sometimes die because of gastrointestinal hemorrhage due to rupture of gastroesophageal varices or hepatic failure with uncontrollable ascites, in spite of good contol of their tumor by means of TAE and/or PEIT [6,7]. Therefore, an important problem in Asian countries is how to treat portal hypertension, variceal hemorrhage, and uncontrollable ascites, as well as how to treat HCC.

Transjugular intrahepatic portosystemic shunt (TIPS) is a new interventional treatment for portal hypertension that was developed by Josef Rosch in 1969 [8] and has been effective in controlling variceal bleeding refractory to endoscopic management, and uncontrollable ascites [9–11]. Because portal hypertension with a liver tumor has previously been considered a contraindication for the procedure [12], TIPS has rarely been applied to patients with hepatocellular carcinoma under the present conditions in Japan, as described above. Between December 1992 and December 1997, we completed the TIPS procedure successfully in 40 of 41 patients, representing a technical success rate of 96%, including 10 patients with hepatocellular carcinoma [13]. We thus believe that TIPS placement can be clinically effective and technically feasible and safe even in patients with HCC. Herein, we review the results of our first ten attempts at placing TIPS in patients with pre-existing HCC and in two patients with incidental occurrence of HCC during observation after TIPS.

Materials and Methods

Patients

Ten of the total of 40 patients who underwent TIPS in our institution already had developed HCC before treatment, and two other patients developed HCC incidentally after TIPS. These 12 patients consisted of either men and four women, ranging in age from 46 to 74 years. Liver disease was classified as Child-Pugh A in ten patients, B in four patients, and C in six patients, with the cause of liver cirrhosis being hepatitis C virus infection in ten patients, and hepatitis B virus infection in ten patients, with no alcoholic causation. Of these 12 patients, 8 were treated electively for uncontrollable ascites, and 4 patients were treated on an emergency basis due to active bleeding from gastroesophageal varices and/or hematemesis at the time of TIPS. In the ten patients with pre-existing HCC, tumors had been well-controlled by TAE and/or PEIT in five, resected in three, and not treated in two patients (Table 1).

TIPS Procedure

The TIPS procedure was essentially the same as that described by Rosch and made use of a coaxial catheter needle system (Cook, Bloomington, IN, USA) [14]. After angiographic and three-dimensional computed tomographic localization of the portal bifurcation, the right hepatic vein was catheterized transjugulary and a coaxial catheter needle system was introduced through a 10-F catheter sheath. Under fluoro-

Table 1. Clinical characteristics of the patients

Patient	Age/Sex	Indication for TIPS	Child-Pugh Classification	Location of tumor	Stent/Diameter	Shunt tract
1.	74/F	Hematoemesis	B	Seg. 6, viable	Z-stent/10 mm	RHV-BIF
2.	58/M	Variceal rupture	B	Seg. 3, 5, controlled	Z-stent/10 mm	RHV-RPV
3.	58/M	Hematoemesis	A	Seg. 5, 8, controlled	Z-stent/10 mm	RHV-RPV
4.	58/F	Variceal rupture	A	Seg. 7–8, controlled	Z-stent/10 mm	RHV-RPV
5.	59/M	Uncontrollable ascites	C	Diffuse, viable	Z-stent/10 mm	RHV-LPV
6.	66/F	Uncontrollable ascites	C	Seg. 3, 5, controlled	Z-stent/10 mm	RHV-RPV
7.	65/M	Uncontrollable ascites	B	Seg. 5, 6, 8, controlled	Z-stent/10 mm	RHV-RPV
8.	50/M	Uncontrollable ascites	C	After resection	Z-stent/10 mm	RHV-RPV
9.	54/F	Uncontrollable ascites	C	After resection	Z-stent/8 mm	RHV-RPV
10.	56/M	Uncontrollable ascites	C	After resection	Wallstent/8 mm	RHV-RPV
11.	58M	Uncontrollable ascites	C	Diffuse (developed after TIPS)	Z-stent/10mm	RHV-RPV
12.	46M	Uncontrollable ascites	C	S8 (developed after TIPS)	Z-stent/10mm	RHV-RPV

TIPS, transjugular intrahepatic portosystemic shunt; RHV, right hepatic vein; RHV, right portal vein; LPV, left portal vein; BIF, bifurcation of portal vein.

scopic guidance, the needle was then advanced, and after puncture of a portal vein branch, a stiff 0.035-inch guide wire was introduced through the needle. A 5-F catheter was advanced into the splenic or mesenteric vein over the guide wire. Portography was performed, and the portal pressures were recorded.

After pressure measurement and portography, the needle tract was dilated with an 8- or 10-mm angioplasty balloon catheter. To create the shunt, an expandable metallic stent was deployed from the portal vein to the hepatic vein. The metallic stents used were Wallstents (Schneider, Minneapolis, MN, USA) in two patients and Modified Z-stents (Cook, Bloomington, IN, USA) in two patients, with a diameter of 8 mm in three patients and 10 mm in nine patients. The TIPS shunt tract originated from the right hepatic vein and bridged to the right portal vein in ten patients, the left hepatic vein in one patient and to the bifurcation of the portal vein in one patient (Table 1). After TIPS placement, portography and measurement of the portosystemic pressure gradient were performed in all patients to test for portal decompression.

Results

Technical Success and Hemodynamic Findings

All of the 12 patients successfully underwent TIPS, a technical success rate of 100%. The number of punctures required to successfully penetrate the portal vein from the hepatic vein was 3.3 on average, with a range of 1–8. Technique-related complications such as tumor rupture, hemobilia, or intraperitoneal hemorrhage were not observed. During the early postprocedural period of 30 days, none of the patients died from a direct complication of the procedure, and the early mortality rate was thus 0%. The mean portosystemic gradient of the 12 patients before successful TIPS was 30.3 mmHg, with a range of 20–41 mmHg. After TIPS, the gradient dropped to an average of 20.4 mmHg, with a range of 15–28 mmHg, an average of 10 mmHg portal decompression (Table 2).

Portograms obtained before stenting in the tract from the hepatic vein to the portal vein revealed hepatofugal blood flow through the left gastric vein, retrogastric vein, short gastric vein, and inferior mesenteric vein, with gastroesophageal varices in 8 of the 12 patients. After TIPS placement, the blood flow through these veins changed to hepatopetal, and the varices disappeared or decreased in all eight patients who had hepatofugal blood flow before the procedure.

Clinical Success

Gastrointestinal hemorrhage due to rupture of gastroesophageal varices refractory to endoscopic sclerotherapy and hematemesis stopped immediately after TIPS in all four patients, and they then recovered from their life-threatening condition. Endoscopically, these varices had completely disappeared in two patients and decreased in size, color, and form in the other two patients.

Table 2. Results

Patient	Portal pressure gradient		Results	Encephalopathy	Shunt occlusion	Outcome/Duration
	Before TIPS	After TIPS				
1.	20 mmHg	→ 15 mmHg	Stopped bleeding	(+)	(−)	Alive 2Y6M
2.	27 mmHg	→ 16 mmHg	Stopped bleeding	(−)	(+)	Alive 2Y6M
3.	38 mmHg	→ 18 mmHg	Stopped bleeding	(−)	(−)	Dead 1Y4M (Tumor)
4.	32 mmHg	→ 24 mmHg	Stopped bleeding	(+)	(−)	Alive 1Y11M
5.	35 mmHg	→ 28 mmHg	No change of ascites	(−)	(+)	Dead 3M (Tumor)
6.	34 mmHg	→ 24 mmHg	No change of ascites	(+)	(−)	Alive 1Y9M
7.	41 mmHg	→ 28 mmHg	Complete disappearance of ascites	(+)	(−)	Dead 2M (Hepatic failure)
8.	28 mmHg	→ 22 mmHg	Complete disappearance of ascites	(−)	(−)	Alive 2Y7M
9.	30 mmHg	→ 27 mmHg	Decrease of ascites	(−)	(−)	Alive 1Y9M
10.	34 mmHg	→ 28 mmHg	No change of ascites	(−)	(−)	Alive 2M
11.	42 mmHg	→ 23 mmHg	Complete disappearance of ascites	(−)	(−)	Dead 2Y7M
12.	28 mmHg	→ 18 mmHg	Complete disappearance of ascites	(+)	(−)	Dead 1Y5M

Y, year(s); M, month(s).

Uncontrollable ascites completely disappeared or decreased in volume in five of the eight patients, as revealed by computed tomograms 1 month after TIPS. However, three patients did not achieve disappearance of the ascites despite good portal decompression after TIPS.

Liver function tests in the early phase up to 1 month after TIPS were unchanged in ten patients, and an increase in the serum bilirubin level was noted in two patients. In one patient, the serum bilirubin level subsequently decreased, and discharge from the hospital was possible 3 months after the procedure. However, another patient died with hepatic failure 2 months later.

Survival

The post-TIPS follow-up periods for the 12 patients ranged from 2–31 months. Seven patients were alive with their tumors stabilized or controlled by TAE and/or PEIT. Five patients died. Of the ten patients with preexisting HCC or who had their tumor resected before the TIPS procedure, three died. Patient no. 3 died after 16 months due to tumor progression and multiple tumor ruptures. Patient no. 5, in whom hepatoma had not been detected by CT scans or angiography and in whom further tumor progression in the right lobe of the liver had already occurred when TIPS was performed, died after 2 months due to tumor progression. Patient no. 7, with severe liver cirrhosis of Child-Pugh class C and uncontrollable ascites, died 2 months after TIPS due to an elevated serum bilirubin level and hepatic failure.

In two patients, no. 11 and no. 12, massive ascites was completely eliminated by means of TIPS, but liver tumors incidentally occurred 29 and 17 months after the procedure. Patient, no. 11 died 31 months after TIPS due to diffuse and rapid growth of tumors. Patient no. 12 died 17 months after TIPS due to acute hepatitis, even though the tumor was small.

Complications

In none of the 12 patients did technique-related complications such as hemobilia, tumor bleeding, or intraperitoneal hemorrhage occur. Hepatic encephalopathy occurred in five patients; this was able to be controlled by lactulose therapy except in one patient who developed hepatic failure 1 month after TIPS. Shunt occlusion occurred in five patients after 1 week and 4, 4.5, and 6 months. Three of these four patients underwent balloon dilatation of the occluded tract, and this resulted in reopening of the shunt and good flow with portal decompression.

Patients

Patient 1

A 74-year-old woman was admitted to our hospital for resection of an HCC which was solitary and encapsulated with exotatic growth in the 6th segment of the liver (Fig. 1a). She also had esophageal varices without any episodes of variceal bleeding

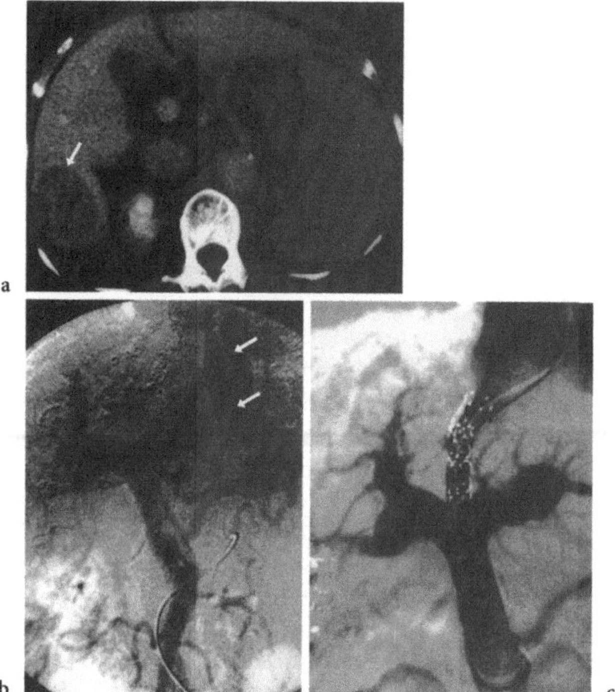

Fig. 1. Patient 1. Images of a 74-year-old female with hepatoma. (a) CT scan before TIPS shows hepatoma with heterogenous density and protruding extension (*arrow*). (b) Venous phase of superior mesenteric arteriogram shows filling of prominent gastroesophageal varices is seen (*arrow*). (c) Portogram obtained after TIPS shows excellent blood flow through the shunt between portal bifrucation and right hepatic vein

(Fig. 1b). While waiting to undergo the resection, variceal rupture occurred and emergency endoscopic sclerotherapy was performed. Although the bleeding from the esophageal varices stopped immediately after the sclerotherapy, hematemesis and anemia continued. Creation of a TIPS was considered because of continuation of hematemesis and anemia in spite of the sclerotherapy. A computed tomography and a hepatic angiography revealed that there was no tumor located in the puncture route from the right hepatic vein to the bifurcation of the portal vein, and TIPS was thus performed. Pressure measurements performed at that time revealed a 20 mm Hg mean gradient between the portal vein and the hepatic vein. A modified Z-stent 10 mm in diameter was deployed in the tract, and portography revealed rapid flow through the shunt and markedly reduced flow into the varices (Fig. 1c). The portosystemic pressure gradient dropped to 15 mmHg. Immediately after TIPS, the hematemesis stopped, and the esophageal varices had completely disappeared on endoscopic observation 1 month after TIPS. She recovered from this serious condition and hepatic embolotherapy was performed 1 month after TIPS, when the liver function had become normal.

Mild, grade I encephalopathy developed for a month and was controlled with lactulose therapy. She had been in her usual state of good health, with no episodes of esophageal rupture and a decrease in the tumor size without recurrence at 2 years and 6 months after the TIPS placement (Fig. 1).

Patient 2

A 58-year-old man experienced multiple episodes of variceal bleeding and underwent endoscopic sclerotherapy. He also had HCCs in the right liver lobe with an episode of tumor rupture; the bleeding had been stopped and was well controlled by multiple hepatic embolotherapies (Fig. 2a).

During the fourth hepatic embolotherapy, rupture of esophageal varices occurred again, and emergency endoscopic sclerotherapy was unsuccessful. TIPS using a modified Z-stent 10mm in diameter was performed and the variceal bleeding was stopped (Fig. 2b). Because of the disappearance of the esophageal varices on endoscopic observation 3 weeks after TIPS, he was discharged from the hospital. However, 2 months later, he entered our hospital again with severe abdominal pain and shock.

A computed tomography revealed two huge tumors and fluid collection around the tumors, suggesting rupture of the tumors, which had been controlled when TIPS was performed 2 months earlier (Fig. 2c). A hepatic angiography also revealed two huge tumors with coarse tumor vessels and extravasation of contrast medium (Fig. 2d). Emergency TAE was successful, and the bleeding from the tumor was completely stopped. He was in good health with patency of the shunt tract and no reccurrent bleeding until 1 year and 3 months after the TIPS placement. Although the tumors had been controlled by three TAEs after TIPS, he died 1 year and 4 months after TIPS of tumor progression and hepatic failure.

Patient 3

A 46-year-old man with marked and rapidly increasing ascites and post—viral Child C cirrhosis was referred for elective TIPS placement. Computed tomography revealed a small liver with an irregular surface and massive ascites (Fig. 3a). A TIPS of 10mm in diameter was placed between the right hepatic vein and the right portal vein (Fig. 3b). The portosystemic pressure gradient was reduced from 27 to 17mmHg, and computed tomography showed no ascites after TIPS. Within 1 month, the abdominal distension disappeared, and he was discharged from the hospital and returned to his job.

For 1 year after TIPS, he was in good health; however, a small tumor in the liver was detected on a follow-up CT scan performed 1 year later (Fig. 3c). Thereafter, he complained of general fatigue and abdominal distension with AST and ALT levels increased to over 500mg/dl. Liver biopsy indicated advanced liver cirrhosis and acute hepatitis. He died 1 year and 5 months after TIPS due to hepatic failure. A postmortem specimen of his liver showed a small HCC in the right lobe of the liver, while the shunt tract was patent and showed slight pseudointimal hyperplasia (Fig. 3d).

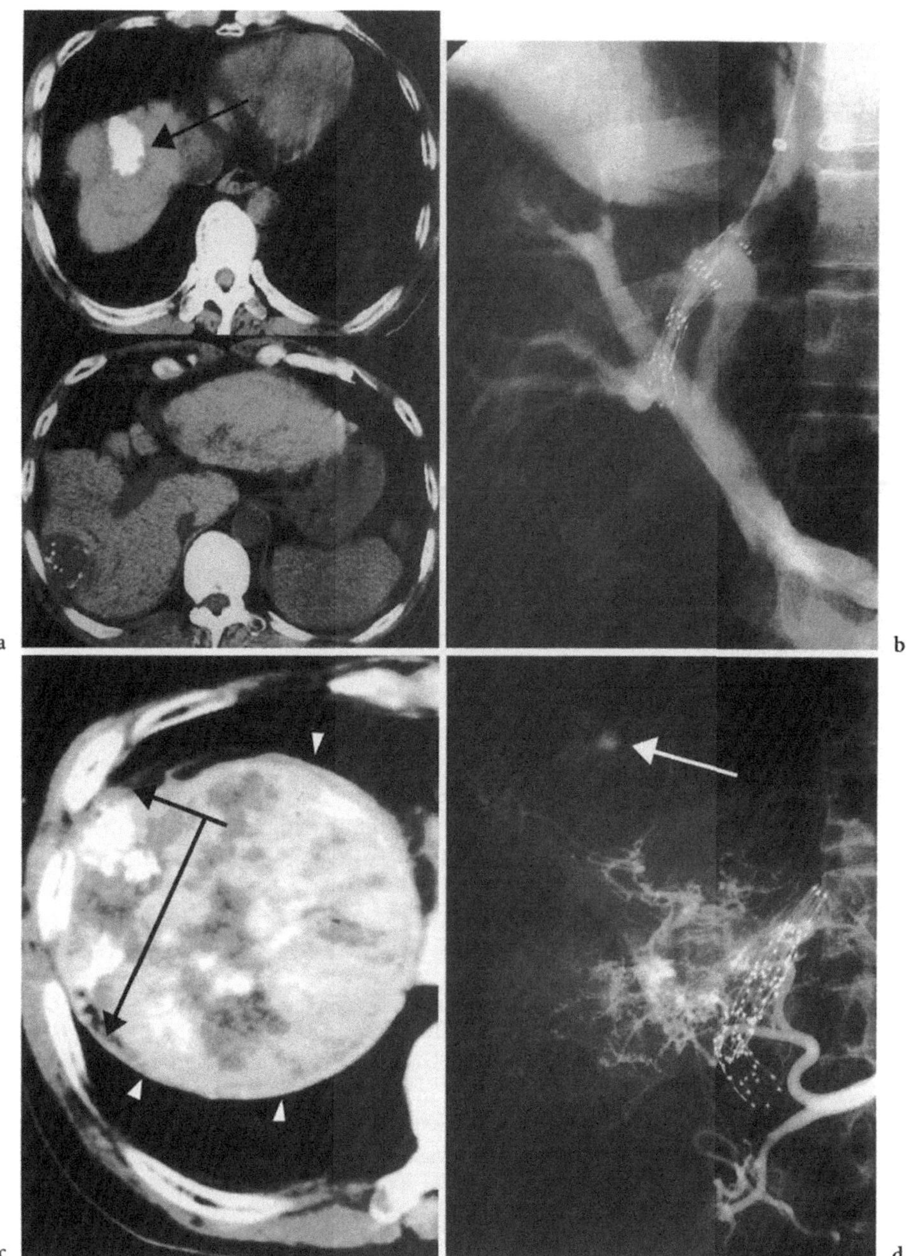

Fig. 2. Patient 2. Images of 58 year-old man with two hepatomas. (**a**) CT scan before TIPS demonstrates tumor with lipiodol accumulation (*arrow*) which has been controlled by mutiple TAEs and PEITs. (**b**) Portal venogram after TIPS placement shows good flow through the shunt. Minimal filling of varices is seen. (**c**) CT scan two month after TIPS shows the tumor remarkably increase in size (*white arrows*) and fluid collection around the tumor, suggested rupture of the tumor (*arrow*). (**d**) Angiogram reveals relative hypovascular tumor with extravasation of contrast media (*arrow*). TAE was performed and stopped bleeding

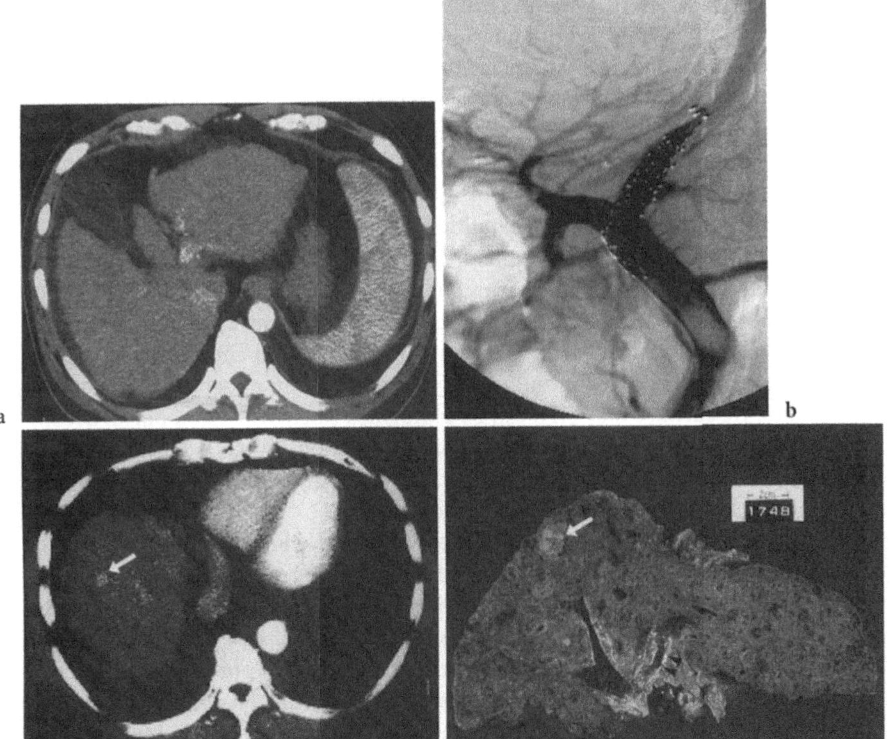

Fig. 3. Patient 3. Images with 46-year old man (**a**) CT scan shows a small liver with irregular margin and massive ascites. Tumor cannot be seen in the liver. (**b**) Portal venogram after TIPS placement using Z-stent 10 mm in diameter reveals exellent flow through the shunt. Portosystemic gradient is reduced from 27 to 17 mmHg. (**c**) Follow-up CT scan 1 year after TIPS placement shows a small tumor (*arrow*). (**d**) Spacemen of the liver in postmorten reveals a small liver tumor (*arrow*) and patent of shunt tract with slight intimal hyperplasia (*arrow heads*)

Discussion

TIPS is an effective treatment for portal hypertension, but TIPS does have some problems, including hepatic encephalopathy, deterioration of liver function, and shunt occlusion after the procedure. Furthermore, the indications and contraindications for TIPS have not been fully established yet, but Rosch stated that a liver tumor was a contraindication for TIPS [12]. This pessimistic outlook has persisted. However, in Japan and other Asian countries, there are some differences from Western countries because of high incidences of liver cirrhosis and portal hypertension due to hepatitis virus infection. HCC occurs especially frequently in hepatitis C virus infection [1–3].

The reported prevalence of HCC in patients with liver cirrhosis and portal hypertension varies widely, and HCC is usually found in over 7% of all patients with hepatitis viral infection for 1 year as reported by the Japanese Liver Cancer Research Group Society [3]. In our series, HCC was present or had been resected in 10 of the 41 patients referred for the TIPS. HCC did not interfere with the TIPS placement.

The therapeutic options for patients with portal hypertension and HCC are limited depending on the extent of the tumor, number of tumors, and liver function. Complications associated with the TIPS procedure have included minor hematomas at the jugular puncture site, chronic shunt occlusion, stent migration, and death secondary to hemorrhage from the transhepatic portal venous tract. In our series of ten patients, who were all in a life-threatening condition and had a poor quality of life due to variceal bleeding refractory to sclerotherapy or uncontrollable ascites, TIPS placement was successful in all cases without technique-related complications.

Furthermore, the results of TIPS were also satisfactory because bleeding completely stopped in all four patients with variceal hemorrhage, and the disappearance or decrease of ascites was observed in four of six patients with massive and uncontrollable ascites. We surmise that TIPS can be performed safely with good portal decompression and recovery from life-threatening conditions such as gastrointestinal hemorrhage and massive ascites, as long as the tumor does not occupy the puncture route and has been controlled by TAE and/or PEIT.

TIPS, however, does alter the hepatic hemodynamics, which may result in hepatic encephalopathy and deterioration of liver function. The reduction or loss of portal liver perfusion that accompanies shunt implantation may also induce a relative increase in arterial liver perfusion. This results in an increase in the hepatic arterial flow, which may possible induce rapid growth of liver tumors pre-existing the procedure and may trigger incidental occurrence of HCC after the procedure. Indeed, two patients developed HCC incidentally during the observation period after TIPS and one patient whose tumors pre-existed but were under control grew rapidly and ruptured only 2 month after the TIPS procedure. However, at present, we cannot draw a conclusion regarding TIPS and incidental occurrence of HCC because of insufficient experience. There may be involvement of the altered hepatic hemodynamics induced by TIPS, or it may be the natural course for patients with hepatitis virus infection. However, we must observe liver tumors carefully by radiological methods at intervals on a long-term basis after TIPS placement because there is a possibility of early tumor progression and rupture.

Our experience with these ten patients indicates that HCC is not necessarily a contraindication to TIPS placement when certain conditions are satisfied: no tumor is located in the puncture route, the tumors are controlled by TAE and/or PEIT, and the portal hypertension is a life-threatening condition such as that associated with variceal rupture and refractory ascites, which is predictive factor for survival.

References

1. Okuda K (1997) Hepatocellular carcinoma: clinicopathological aspects. J Gastroenterol Hepatol 12(9–10):S314–318
2. Chen CH, et al. (1998) Characteristics of hepatocellular carcinoma presenting with variceal bleeding. J Gastroenterol Hepatol 13(2):170–174

3. Oka H, Kurioka N, Kanno T (1990) Prospective detection of hepatocellular carcinoma in patients with cirrhosis. Hepatology 12:680–687
4. Yamada R, Sato M, Kawabata M (1983) Hepatic artery embolization in 120 patients with hepatoma. Radiology 148:397–401
5. Matsui O, Kadoya M, Yoshikawa J (1993) Small hepatocellular carcinoma: Treatment with subsegmental transcatheter arterial embolization. Radiology 188:79–83
6. Nomura H, et al. (1999) Rebamipide prevents occurrence of gastric lesions following transcatheter arterial embolization in the hepatic artery. J Gastroenterol Hepatol 14(5):495–499
7. Bianco S, et al. (1996) Short-term effects of transcatheter arterial chemoembolisation on metabolic activity of the liver of cirrhotic patients with hepatocellular carcinoma. Gut 39(2):325–329
8. Rosch J, Hanafee WN, Snow H (1969) Transjugular portal venography and radiologic portocaval shunt: an experience study. Radiology 92:588–592
9. LaBerge JM (1991) Transjugular intrahepatic portosystemic shunt with the Wallstent expandable metallic endoprosthesis. JVIR 16:258–267
10. Ring EJ, Lake JR, Roberts AP (1992) Percutaneous intrahepatic portosystemic shunts to control variceal bleeding prior to liver transplantation. Ann Intern Med 116:304–309
11. Yamada R, Sato M, Kishi K (1992) Nippon Acta Radiol 52:1328–1330
12. Rosch J, Barton RE, Keller FS, et al. (1992) Transjugular Intrahepatic Portosystemic Shunt. Probl Surg 9:502–512
13. Nakamura K, et al. (1995) Transjugular intrahepatic portosystemic shunt for patients with hepatoma (in Japanese). Nippon Igaku Hoshasen Gakkai Zasshi 55(3):187–189
14. Uchida B, Putnam J, Buschman R (1987) A traumatic transjugular needle for portal vein puncture in swine. Radiology 163:580–581
15. Richter GM, Noeldge G, Palmaz JC (1991) The transjugular intrahepatic portosystemic stent-shunt (TIPSS): results of a pilot study. Cardiovasc Intervent Radiol 13:200–207
16. Zemel G, Katzen BT, Becker GJ (1991) Percutaneous transjugular portosystemic shunt. JAMA 266:309–393
17. Hauenstein KH, Haag K, Ochs A (1995) The reducing stent: Treatment for transjugular intrahepatic portosystemic shunt-induced refractory hepatic encephalopathy and liver failure. Radiology 194:175–179
18. Burchell AR, Rousselot LM, Panke WF (1968) A seven-year experience with side-to-side portocaval shunt for cirrhotic ascites. Ann Surg 168:655–670

Prevention of Hepatocarcinogenesis by Fibrosuppression

Isao Sakaida, Koji Hironaka, and Kiwamu Okita

Summary. A choline-deficient L-amino acid-defined (CDAA) diet led to the development of liver cirrhosis in 100% of male Wistar rats after 15 weeks and liver neoplasms in 90% of rats after one year. Concurrent administration of a prolyl 4-hydroxylase inhibitor (HOE 077) [2,4-pyridine dicarboxylic acid bis (2-methoxyethylamide)] at a dose of 200 ppm as an antifibrotic agent to rats fed a CDAA diet reduced the increase in liver hydroxyproline content without reduction of serum ALT. HOE 077 prevented the activation of stellate cells, as determined histologically, as well as the expression of procollagen type I mRNA, resulting in reduced hydroxyproline levels in the liver. Also, the administration of a CDAA diet for 15 weeks led to a substantial induction of GSTP-positive lesions and the production of 8-hydroxydeoxyguanosine (8OHdG) in the liver. The concurrent administration of HOE 077 reduced the area of GSTP-positive lesions, in parallel with the reduction in hydroxyproline content. Administration of HOE 077 for 1 year reduced the development of liver neoplasms to 50% of rats fed a CDAA diet with reduced hydroxyproline and 8OHdG content. These data suggest that inhibition of fibrosis may prevent the development of neoplasms.

Key words. Fibrosis, Carcinogenesis, Prolyl 4-hydroxylase inhibitor, Enzyme-altered lesions, Stellate cell

Introduction

Hepatocellular carcinoma is usually associated with liver cirrhosis, mainly as a consequence of chronic hepatitis or alcohol consumption, although the relationships between carcinogenesis and fibrosis (liver cirrhosis) are unknown.

There have been two basic approaches to the prevention of liver cancer. The first approach is causation prevention, in which causative agents are eliminated or reduced. Hepatitis, alcohol, and aflatoxins are major causes which have been identified, and the prevention of liver cancer by the elimination of such causes has considerable poten-

First Department of Internal Medicine, School of Medicine, Yamaguchi University, 1144 Kogushi, Ube, Yamaguchi 755-8505, Japan

tial. The second approach is interventional prevention, in which a protective agent, either chemical (chemoprevention) or biological, is administered to prevent or reduce carcinogenesis. In situations where the causes are unknown or cannot be completely eliminated, such as in chronic hepatitis B or C, only interventional prevention is available. There have been many reports concerning the prevention of liver cancer in rodents by butylated hydroxytoluene (BHT), retinoids, S-adenosyl-L-methionine, and other agents [1,2]. But in clinical practice there has been no effective agent for chemoprevention so far.

Thus, in the present study, we examined the effect of prolyl 4-hydroxylase inhibitor (HOE 077) [2,4-pyridine dicarboxylic acid bis (2-methoxyethylamide)] on the development of enzyme-altered lesions of glutathione S-transferase placental form (GSTP) (preneoplastic lesions) and DNA damage (as measured by 8-hydroxydeoxyguanosine [8OHdG] production) in rat liver cirrhosis induced by the administration of a CDAA diet for 15 weeks [3]. The effects of HOE 077 on the development of hepatocellular carcinoma induced by the administration of a CDAA diet for 52 weeks were also examined. Our data suggest that inhibition of fibrosis (liver cirrhosis) may prevent the development of liver neoplasms and this represents a new approach for the prevention of liver neoplasms.

Materials and Methods

Animals

Male Wistar rats 6 weeks of age and weighing 140–150g (Nippon SLC, Shizuoka, Japan) were obtained, quarantined for 1 week, and housed in a room under controlled temperature (25°C), humidity, and lighting (12h light, 12h dark). Access to food and tap water was ad libitum throughout the study period. After a 1-week acclimation period on a basal diet (Oriental MF Diet, Oriental Yeast, Japan), the rats were divided into experimental groups.

Diets

The CDAA and choline supplemented L-amino acid-defined (CSAA) diets were obtained in powdered form (Dyets, Bethlehem, PA, USA; product numbers 518753, 518754). The detailed compositions of these diets have been described in a previous report [4].

A prolyl 4-hydroxylase inhibitor (HOE 077) 2,4-pyridine dicarboxylic acid bis (2-methoxyethylamide) (Hoechst, Frankfurt, Germany) in powdered form (MW 281, white powder, melting point 86°C, soluble in water, purity more than 99.9%) was mixed evenly into the CDAA diet.

Experimental Protocol

The total study periods were 15 or 52 weeks. The groups for assessing the effect of HOE 077 on hydroxyproline content (15-week experiment) consisted of 10 or 3 rats each. Two groups of 10 rats received a CDAA diet with HOE 077 at a concentrations of 200 or 0 ppm. One group of 3 rats received a CSAA diet as a control. For the experiment on liver neoplasm development, two groups of 10 rats received a CDAA diet with or without 200 ppm HOE 077 for 52 weeks.

At the end of the study, all rats were killed under ether anesthesia. Blood was obtained from the bifurcation of the abdominal aorta and the liver was excised. The livers were weighed, then immediately frozen for hydroxyproline measurements or fixed and embedded in paraffin as described previously [5].

Histology and Immunohistochemical Examination

Sections of 5-μm thickness of the right lobe of all rat livers were processed routinely for hematoxylin and eosin and Azan-Mallory staining and examined immunohistochemically for α smooth muscle actin (α SMA), glutathione-S-transferase placental form (GSTP), and 8-hydroxydeoxyguanosine (8HOdG) by the advidin–biotin–peroxidase-complex method as previously described [6]. Anti-αSMA monoclonal antibody (DAKO, Kyoto, Japan), rabbit anti-rat GSTP antibody (MBL, Nagoya, Japan), and anti-8OHdG monoclonal antibody (Nihon-Yushi, Tokyo, Japan) were used [6,7]. Quantitative analysis of GSTP-positive lesions was then carried out with an image analysis system (Personal Image Analysis System LA-555, Pias, Osaka, Japan). The area of GSTP-positive lesions was expressed as a percentage of the total area of the specimen as described previously [4,5]. The incidence of hepatocellular carcinomas was assessed by macroscopic findings. The suspected lesions were excised and confirmed by histological examination.

Hydroxyproline Content. Hydroxyproine content was determined by the modified Kivirikko's method as previously described [5].

Probes. The following probes were used in this study. The complementary deoxynucleic acid (cDNA) of type I procollagen alpha 2 and G3PDH (glyceraldehyde-3-phosphate dehydrogenase) were used [8].

Northern Blot Analysis. Northern blot analysis was performed after isolation of total RNA from the liver tissue by extraction of guanidine isothiocyanate as described previously [8].

8OHdG Measurement. The amount of 8OHdG was measured by the methods previously reported [3].

Statistical Methods. Results are expressed as the mean ± SD, and the data were evaluated by ANOVA as was appropriate. The level of significance was set at $P < .05$ for each analysis.

Results

Table 1 indicates that rats fed a CDAA diet for 15 weeks showed an increased liver hydroxyproline content of $753 \pm 102\,\mu g/g$ wet weight, compared with $136 \pm 57\,\mu g/g$ wet weight for rats fed a CSAA diet. Concurrent administration of HOE 077 at 200 ppm significantly reduced this increase in hydroxyproline content to $538 \pm 123\,\mu g/g$ wet weight.

HOE 077 at 200 ppm prevented the formation of pseudolobuli and reduced the thickness of fibrous septa seen by light microscopy (Fig. 1), in parallel with the reduction in the hydroxyproline content of the liver (Table 1). Administration of HOE 077 (200 ppm) did not notably change the histological findings other than the reduced formation of fibrous septa, e.g., liver cell necrosis or fatty changes, which may have influenced the development of enzyme-altered lesions. The inhibition of fibrosis by HOE 077 cannot be attributed to the reduced cell damage because HOE 077 did not reduce the increased serum ALT level of rats fed a CDAA diet.

Activated stellate cells that express αSMA are called myofibroblast-like cells and are now considered the main collagen producing cells. These cells markedly proliferated in the liver of rats fed a CDAA diet for 15 weeks (Fig. 2A). HOE 077 at 200 ppm again reduced the number of αSMA-positive cells in the liver (Fig. 2B). Thus, the prevention of fibrogenesis by HOE 077 is somehow related to the inhibition of activation of stellate cells. Hepatocyte nuclei were also positive for 8OHdG in the livers of rats fed a CDAA diet for 15 weeks (Fig. 3).

α_2(I) Procollagen transcript was clearly demonstrated by the Northern blot analysis of poly $(A)^+$ RNA isolated from the livers of the rats fed the CDAA diet alone or with 200 ppm of HOE 077 for 15 weeks. The levels of α_2(I) procollagen mRNA expression clearly decreased in the livers of rats fed a CDAA diet with 200 ppm HOE 077 for 15 weeks (Fig. 4). Thus, the prevention of fibrosis by HOE 077 can be attributed not only to the inhibition of hydroxylation of the proline but also to the prevention of stellate cell activation resulting in reduced gene expression of procollagen.

Typical GSTP-positive nodules surrounded by fibrous septa are shown in Fig. 5. In this model at 15 weeks, GSTP-positive lesions are mainly consist of these nodules.

Table 1. Effect of HOE 077 on various markers after the 15-week experiment

Treatment (number of rats)	Hydroxyproline ($\mu g/g$ wet wt)	GSTP-positive lesions (%)	ALT (U/L)
CDAA (10)	753 ± 102	5.88 ± 2.11	253 ± 67
+HOE 077/200 ppm (10)	$*538 \pm 123$	$**3.63 \pm 1.75$	282 ± 65
CSAA (3)	136 ± 57	—	53 ± 8

Each number represents mean $\pm$ SD.

GSTP, glutathione S-transferase placental form; CDAA, choline-deficient L-amino acid-defined; CSAA, choline-supplemented L-amino acid-defined (CDAA) diet; HOE 077, 2,4-pyridine dicarboxylic acid bis (2-methoxyethylamide).

$*P < .01$ versus CDAA group.

$**P < .05$ versus CDAA group.

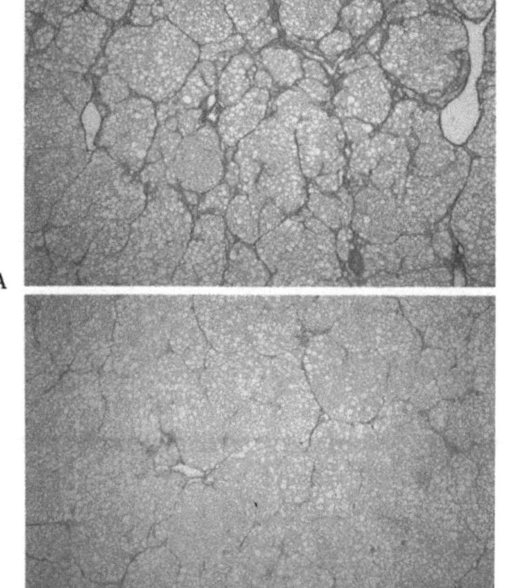

Fig. 1. Photomicrograph of a liver section stained with Azan-Mallory from a male Wistar rat fed a choline-deficient L-amino acid-defined (CDAA) diet for 15 weeks (**A**), and from a rat fed a CDAA diet with concomitant administration of 200 ppm of HOE 077 for 15 weeks (**B**). ×40

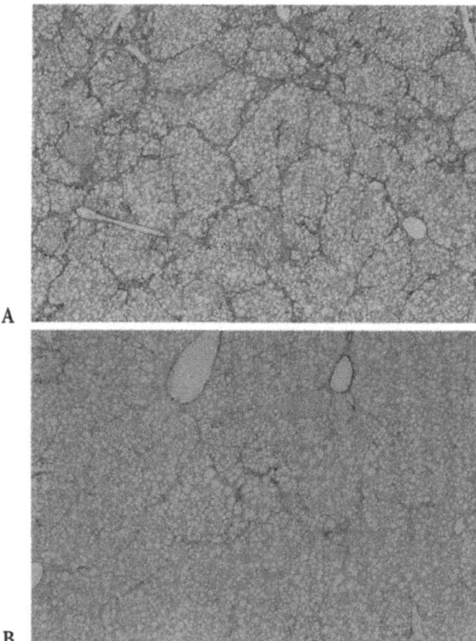

Fig. 2. Photomicrographs of liver sections stained with anti-rat α-smooth muscle actin antibody from a male Wistar rat fed a CDAA diet for 15 weeks (**A**) from a rat fed a CDAA diet with concomitant administration of 200 ppm of HOE 077 for 15 weeks (**B**). ×40

Fig. 3. Photomicrograph of liver sections stained with anti-8-hydroxydeoxyguanosine (8OHdG) antibody from a male Wistar rat fed a CDAA diet for 15 weeks. ×100

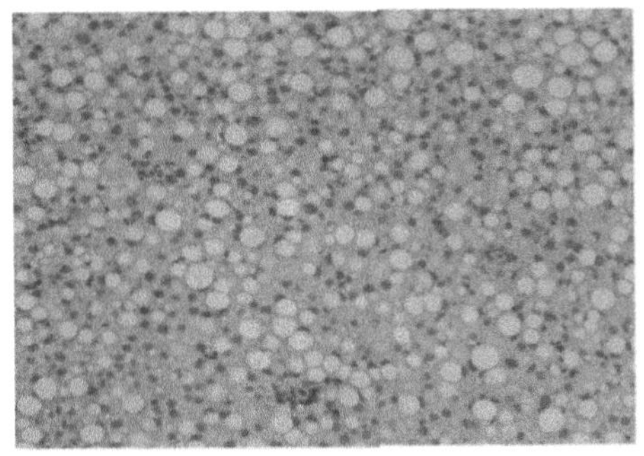

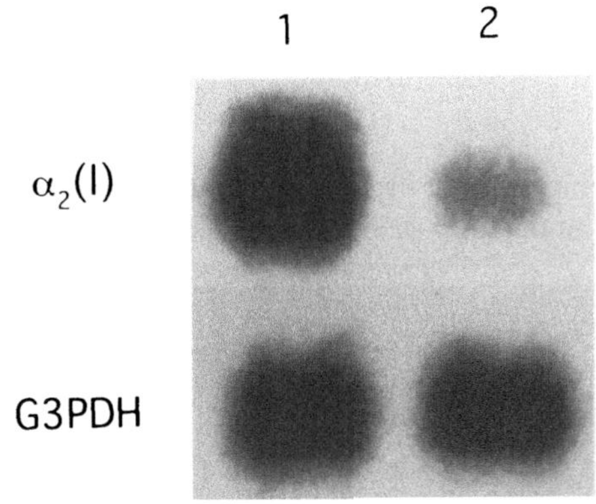

Fig. 4. Messenger RNA expression of α_2 (I) procollagen and G3PDH in the livers of rats fed a CDAA diet alone (*lane 1*) or a CDAA diet with 200 ppm of HOE 077 for 15 weeks (*lane 2*). The figure shows a representative example of 5 independent Northern blots

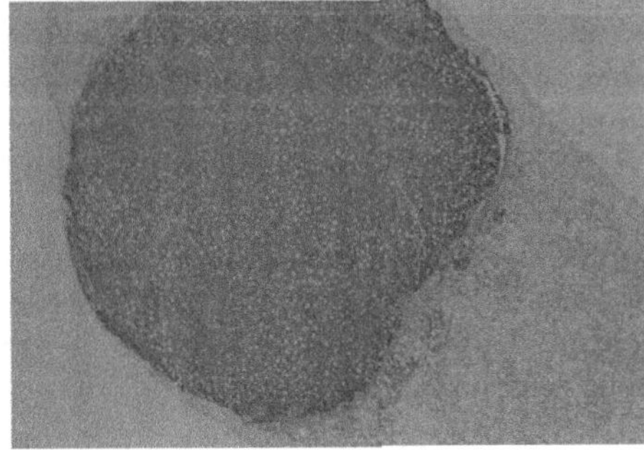

Fig. 5. Typical photomicrograph of GSTP-positive nodules surrounded by fibrous septa in a liver section from a male Wistar rat fed a CDAA diet for 15 weeks. ×40

The results of quantitative analysis of GSTP-positive lesions of the liver at the end of the study are also summarized in Table 1. A CDAA diet for 15 weeks was associated with the development of a large number of GSTP-positive lesions. The concomitant administration of HOE 077 significantly reduced such lesions in a dose-dependent manner, in parallel with the reduced hydroxyproline content.

The administration of a CDAA diet for 52 weeks induced the development of hepatocellular carcinomas in 90% of rats (Fig. 6). HOE 077 at 200 ppm reduced the

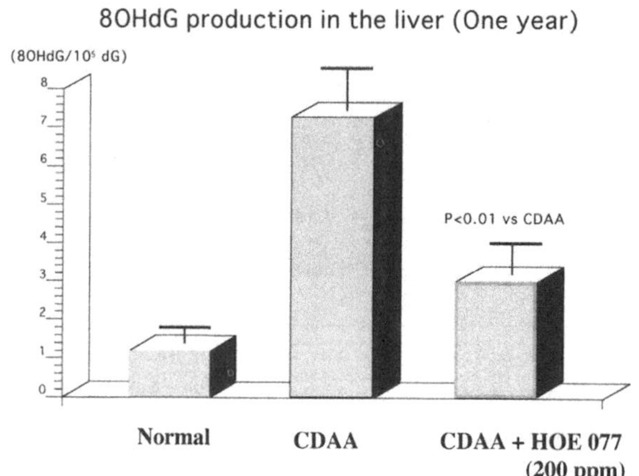

Fig. 6. Comparison of 8-hydroxydeoxyguanosine (8OHdG) production in the livers of rats fed a CDAA or a CSAA (*normal*) diet for 52 weeks with or without 200 ppm HOE 077

incidence of liver neoplasms to 50% of rats. Also, HOE 077 reduced significantly the amount of 8OHdG in noncancerous lesions of the liver as shown in Fig. 6.

Discussion

Using rat liver fibrosis induced by a CDAA diet, the effects of a prolyl 4-hydroxylase inhibitor (HOE 077) on the development of preneoplastic lesions and neoplasms of the liver were investigated.

HOE 077 is designed as a prodrug. In its original state, it is not an effective inhibitor of prolyl 4-hydroxylase, but it is able to cross biological membranes. It is well absorbed from the gastrointestinal tract and is taken up by the liver, where it is converted to active metabolites which are competitive inhibitors of prolyl 4-hydroxylase within the hepatocytes [9]. Also in primary human and rat hepatocytes, HOE 077 is effective in preventing the hydroxylation of proline in a dose-dependent manner [10]. The inhibition of prolyl 4-hydroxylase results in the formation of underhydroxylated collagen species that are not able to form the stable triple helix of procollagen molecules, and are then rapidly degraded.

Stellate cells are now considered the main collagen-producing cell under nonphysiological conditions [11] and also in our experimental model [12]. As already mentioned, the prolyl 4-hydroxylase inhibitor HOE 077 is a hydrophobic prodrug which can be converted to active hydrophilic metabolites only within hepatocytes, and the effect of fibrosuppression was proven to be liver-specific [13].

Our results indicate that HOE 077 reduced the liver hydroxyproline levels in rats fed a CDAA diet. A CDAA diet alone dramatically increased the hydroxyproline content of the liver by a factor of more than 7 times, compared with a CSAA diet. The administration of 200 ppm HOE 077 was found to cause an almost 30% inhibition of this hydroxyproline accumulation without reducing the increased serum ALT level

(Table 1). Thus, the inhibition of fibrosis by HOE 077 cannot be attributed to the direct action of preventing liver cell death.

Histologically, a reduced number of pseudolobuli and incomplete formation of pseudolobuli, as well as thinner fibrous septa were found, in accordance with the reduced hydroxyproline content of the liver. These results indicate that this prolyl 4-hydroxylase inhibitor effectively retarded the development of liver cirrhosis in rats fed a CDAA diet. However the mechanism of prevention of liver fibrosis seems to be different from that expected by the character of this drug as a prolyl 4-hydroxylase inhibitor.

Research by Wu et al. [14] suggested a mechanism of fibrosuppression by HOE 077, whereby the COOH or NH_2 terminal propeptides of collagen inhibit the synthesis of collagen in culture or cell-free systems. These findings are the same as ours in part and suggest posttranscriptional downregulation. Our results indicate that a prolyl 4-hydroxylase inhibitor can prevent fibrosis by inhibiting not only the hydroxylation of proline but also the expression of procollagen mRNA, presumably by inhibiting the activation of stellate cells.

The sequence of cellular changes in the liver proceeds from hepatocytes to enzyme-altered foci and then to hepatocellular neoplasms [15]. Thus, the induction of enzyme-altered foci or nodules can serve as an indicator of preneoplastic change. Especially, GSTP-positive lesions have been used as a marker of preneoplastic lesions [16]. In addition, the extent of GSTP-positive lesions was in parallel with the generation of 8OHdG in DNAs (Fig. 3) as a result of continuous free-radical-associated DNA damage by the CDAA diet [3].

At 15 weeks with a CDAA diet alone, GSTP-positive lesions mainly consisted of nodules surrounded by fibrous septa, resulting in the formation of pseudolobuli (Fig. 5). HOE 077 reduced the area of GSTP-positive lesions. The inhibition of the formation of GSTP-positive lesions by this antifibrous agent is consistent with the reduction in the hydroxyproline content of the liver. The liver hydroxyproline content reflects the number of collagen fibers making up the fibrous septa [17]. Therefore, the inhibition of GSTP-positive lesions by HOE 077 can be presumed to be attributable to the prevention of pseudolobule formation by fibrous septa. Also, it has been reported that the extent of GSTP-positive lesions parallels the generation of 8OHdG in DNA, which appears to be the major molecular effect caused by a CDAA diet [3].

Our 52-week experiment indicates that fibrosuppression may prevent the development of liver neoplasms (Table 2). Fibrosuppression reduced DNA damage (8OHdG production) in the liver caused by oxitative stress as shown in Fig. 6, although the mechanism is unknown.

Table 2. Incidence of hepatocellular carcinomas (HCC) after the 52-week experiment

Treatment	CDAA	CDAA + 200 ppm HOE 077
Number of rats	10	10
Incidence of HCC	90%	50%

CDAA, choline-deficient L-amino acid-defined; HOE 077, 2,4-pyridine dicarboxylic acid bis (2-methoxyethylamide).

Recently, we have reported that pre-exisiting fibrosis induced by pig serum injection without hepatocyte injury and regeneration accelerates GSTP-positive lesion formation under a CDAA diet [18]. However, as the mechanism of cancer prevention by fibrosuppression is still obscure, further research is necessary. Thus, the main result of the present study is that there was at least some correlation between fibrosis and preneoplastic lesions/liver neoplasms.

Clinically useful chemoprevention has not yet been established; therefore, the prevention of fibrosis constitutes a new approach for the prevention of liver neoplasms.

References

1. Williams GM, Tanaka T, Maruyama H, Maeura Y, Weisburg JH, Zang E (1982) Modulation by butylated hydroxytoluene of liver and bladder carcinogenesis induced by chronic low-level exposure to 2-acetylaminofluorene. Cancer Res 51:6224–6230
2. Hill DL, Grubbs CJ (1992) Retinoids and cancer prevention. Annu Rev Nutr 12:161–181
3. Yoshiji H, Nakae D, Mizumoto Y, Horiguchi K, Tamura K, Denda A, Tsuji T, Konishi Y (1992) Inhibitory effect of dietary iron deficiency on inductions of putative preneoplastic lesions as well as 8-hydroxydeoxyguanosine in DNA and lipid peroxidation in the livers of rats caused by exposure to a choline-deficient L-amino acid defined diet. Carcinogenesis 13:1227–1233
4. Sakaida I, Matsumura Y, Kubota M, Kayano K, Takenaka K, Mori K, Okita K (1996) The prolyl 4-hydroxylase inhibitor (HOE 077) prevents activation of Ito cells, reducing procollagen gene expression in rat liver fibrosis induced by choline-deficient L-amino acid-defined diet. Hepatology 23:755–763
5. Sakaida I, Kubota M, Kayano K, Takenaka K, Mori K, Okita K (1994) Prevention of fibrosis reduces enzyme-altered lesions in the rat liver. Carcinogenesis 15:2201–2206
6. Sakaida I, Matsumura Y, Akiyama S, Hayashi K, Ishige A, Okita K (1998) Herbal medicine Sho-saiko-to (TJ-9) prevents liver fibrosis and enzyme-altered lesions in rat liver cirrhosis induced by a choline-deficient L-amino acid-defined diet. J Hepatol 28:298–306
7. Sakaida I, Uchida K, Matsumura Y, Okita K (1998) Interferon gamma treatment prevents procollagen gene expression without affecting TGF-β1 expression in pig serum-induced rat liver fibrosis. J Hepatol 28:471–479
8. Matsumura Y, Sakaida I, Uchida K, Kimura T, Ishihara T, Okita K (1997) Prolyl 4-hydroxylase inhibitor (HOE 077) inhibits pig serum-induced rat liver fibrosis by preventing stellate cell activation. J Hepatol 27:185–192
9. Hanauske-Abel HM (1991) Prolyl 4-hydroxylase, a target enzyme for drug development: Design of suppressive agents and the in vitro effects of inhibitors and proinhibitors. J Hepatol 13(Suppl. 3):S8–S16
10. Clement B, Chesne C, Satie AP, Guillouzo A (1991) Effects of the prolyl 4-hydroxylase proinhibitor HOE 077 on human and rat hepatocytes in primary culture. J Hepatol 13(Suppl. 3):S41–S47
11. Friedman SL (1993) The cellular basis of hepatic fibrosis. N Engl J Med 328:1828–1835
12. Sakaida I (1996) Hepatic fibrogenesis and carcinogenesis. Bull Yamaguchi Med Sch 43:45–48

13. Bickel M, Baader E, Brocks DG, Brocks DG, Engelbart K, Gunzer V, Schmids HL, Vogel GH (1991) Beneficial effects of inhibitors of prolyl 4-hydroxylase in CCl_4-induced fibrosis of the liver in rats. J Hepatol 13(Suppl. 3): S26–S34
14. Wu CH, Donovan CB, Wu GY (1986) Evidence for pretranslational regulation of collagen synthesis by procollagen propeptides. J Biol Chem 261:10482–10484
15. Kitahara A, Satoh K, Nishimura K, Ishikawa T, Ruike K, Sato K, Tsuda H, Ito N (1984) Changes in molecular forms of rat hepatic glutathione S-transferase during chemical hepatocarcinogenesis. Cancer Res 44:2698–2703
16. Satoh K, Kitahara A, Soma Y, Inaba Y, Hatayama I, Sato K (1985) Purification, induction and distribution of placental glutathione transferase: A new marker enzyme for preneoplastic cells in chemical hepatocarcinogenesis in the rat. Proc Natl Acad Sci USA 82:3964–3968
17. Nakano M (1986) Morphogenesis of septa in hepatic fibrosis induced by choline deficiency in rats. Acta Pathol Jpn 36:1643–1652
18. Sakaida I, Hironaka K, Uchida K, Suzuki C, Kayano K, Okita K (1998) Fibrosis accelerates the development of enzyme-altered lesions in the rat liver. Hepatology 28:1247–1252

Cancer Vaccination by B7-1-Transfected Hepatocellular Carcinoma Cells

Tomohide Tatsumi, Tetsuo Takehara, Yutaka Sasaki, Masatsugu Hori, and Norio Hayashi

Summary. Human hepatocellular carcinoma (HCC), one of the most common cancers, frequently recurs after primary therapy. A way to prevent this recurrence is needed. Enhanced immunity to some experimental tumors has been observed after transfection of the gene encoding the costimulatory molecule B7-1, a ligand for the CD28/cytolytic T-lymphocyte-associated antigen (CTLA) -4 counter receptor. However, it is not known whether the transfection of B7-1 gene into HCC cells could be useful for HCC treatment. To assess this, we introduced the B7-1 (CD80) gene into HCC cells. We investigated the expressions of B7-1, B7-2, and human leukocyte antigen (HLA) class I in seven human hepatocellular carcinoma (HCC) cell lines by flow cytometric analysis. Flow cytometric analysis revealed that they all expressed B7-1, B7-2, and HLA class I on the cell surface. However, the expression levels of B7-1 and B7-2 were very low while those of HLA class I were high. By human transfecting HCC cells with a plasmid containing human B7-1 cDNA, we were able to establish HCC cell lines strongly expressing B7-1. From mixed lymphocyte and tumor culture analysis, the primary cytolytic activity against parental HCC cells could be induced effectively by B7-1-transfected HCC cells. Furthermore, in the mouse tumor model, we found that overexpression of B7-1 on tumor cells can inhibit subcutaneous tumor development in syngeneic BALB/c mice. Vaccination with B7-1-transfected mouse HCC cells was effective as a tumor vaccine for preventing tumor development of parental HCC cells, and splenocytes from mice immunized with B7-1-transfected HCC cells showed cytolytic activity against parental HCC cells. Theses results demonstrate that vaccination of B7-1-transfected HCC cells can induce systemic immunity against parental HCC cells and suggest that vaccination of B7-1-transfected HCC cells may be therapeutically useful for suppressing HCC recurrence.

Key words. Hepatocellular carcinoma, B7-1, Immunization, Gene therapy, Antitumor immunity

---

Department of Internal Medicine and Therapeutics, and Department of Molecular Therapeutics, Osaka University Graduate School of Medicine, 2-2 Yamadaoka, Suita, Osaka 565-0871, Japan

Introduction

The induction of T-cell responses is believed to depend on two combined signals provided by antigen-presenting cells (APC): one is the interaction of T-cell receptors with antigen on the major histocompatibility complex (MHC), and the other is delivered by costimulatory molecules through their counter-receptors on the T lymphocytes [1–4]. In the absence of costimulation, T-cell receptor–antigen interactions appear to induce an anergic state in T cells [5,6]. Recently, B7 family ligands [B7-1 [7–11] and B7-2 [12–16]) for CD28/cytolytic T-lymphocyte-associated antigen (CTLA) -4 have been identified as important costimulatory molecules for inducing antigen-specific major histocompatability (MHC) restricted T-cell activation. The B7-1 or B7-2 molecules are strongly expressed on professional APCs such as activated B cells, macrophages, and dendritic cells [10,11,16].

Costimulation mediated by B7-1 and B7-2 plays an important role in the induction of T-cell-mediated antitumor immunity [17–23]. By transfection of the murine B7-1 gene into mouse tumor cells, protective and sometimes curative immunity against wild-type tumors has been induced in several mouse models [18–22]. Murine melanoma cells transfected with the B7-1 gene were able to induce rejection of non-transfected melanoma in vivo by CD8$^+$ T cells [19]. Recently, it has been demonstrated that B7-2-transfected mastocytoma cells can also induce CD8$^+$ T-cell-mediated tumor immunity similar to that previously observed for B7-1 [23]. Thus, B7-1 and B7-2 expression on tumor cells is thought to be important for generation of antitumor immunity.

Human hepatocellular carcinoma (HCC) is one of the most common cancers. Although HCC patients undergo medical and surgical treatment, intrahepatic and extrahepatic recurrence frequently occurs. Augmentation of antitumor immunity against HCC should afford a new therapeutic method. In previous studies, expression of MHC and intercellular adhesion molecule-1 (ICAM-1) on HCC cells has been thought to participate in the antitumor immune response against human HCC [24,25]. However, the role, if any, of B7-1 and B7-2 expression on HCC cells in antitumor immunity remains unclear.

In the present study, we examined whether B7-1 and B7-2 are expressed in human HCC cell lines by using RT-PCR and flow cytometry and evaluated the regulation of cytokines such as IFN-α, IFN-γ and IL-12. The results suggested that the expression levels of B7-1 and B7-2 on human HCC cells were low but could be increased by interferons (IFNs) [26]. We also tried to establish an HCC cell line that strongly expressed B7-1 by transfecting the human B7-1 gene into human HCC cells and evaluated the role of B7-1 expression in the induction of primary cytolytic activity against human HCC [26]. Moreover, we established an HCC cell line that strongly expressed B7-1 by transfecting the mouse B7-1 gene into poorly immunogenic mouse HCC cells and examined whether it could induce antitumor immunity in vivo.

Materials and Methods

Mice

Female BALB/c mice were purchased from Shizuoka Experimental Animal Laboratory (Shizuoka, Japan) and used at 6–8 weeks of age. All animals were maintained in microisolator cages and handled under aseptic conditions. Procedures were performed according to approved protocols and in accordance with recommendations for the proper care and use of laboratory animals.

Cell Lines and Cell Culture

For the in vitro experiments, we used seven human HCC cell lines (Hep3B, HepG2, Huh-6, Huh-7, HB611, PLC/PRF/5, and KYN-3). RAJI, a human Burkitt lymphoma cell line, and H4IIEC3, a rat HCC cell line, were purchased from ATCC (Rockville, MD, USA). For in vivo study, the murine BNL 1ME A.7R.1 HCC cell line (BNL), which is adherent and was originally established from BALB/c mice, was used.

Flow Cytometry

We investigated the expression of surface B7-1, B7-2, and HLA class I on HCC cell lines with or without cytokine treatments (human IFN-α, 1–1 000 U/ml; human IFN-γ, 1–1 000 U/ml; and human IL-12, 0.1–10 ng/ml) using flow cytometry. We used anti-human B7-1 monoclonal antibody/biotin (Ancell, Bayport, MN, USA), anti-human B7-2 monoclonal antibody/biotin (Pharmingen, San Diego, CA, USA), and anti-HLA-ABC monoclonal antibody (Serotec, Oxford, UK). Flow cytometry was performed using a FACScan system (Becton Dickinson, San Jose, CA, USA). The expressions of B7-1 and B7-2 on human HCC cells were examined with the positive cell rate (%) determined by using cells labeled with the isotype antibody as a control. These experiments were repeated twice and the mean values were analyzed. The induction of B7-1 and B7-2 by cytokines was evaluated from the stimulation index (S.I., mean fluorescence intensity of cytokine-treated cells/mean fluorescence intensity of untreated cells). We regarded the results as upregulation of B7-1 and B7-2 molecule expressions from control experiments if increases of more than 1.28 and 1.41 (the mean value + 10 SD) respectively, were found in the S.I.

Induction of Primary Cytolytic Activity In Vitro

To establish HCC cells strongly expressing B7-1, Hep3B was transfected with the pBJ-human B7-1 expression vector. B7-1 expression was evaluated by flow cytometry. Peripheral blood mononuclear cells (PBMC) (5×10^6) were cocultured with mitomycin-C-treated transfected Hep3B cells (5:1 responder to tumor cell ratio) or with mitomycin-C-treated parental Hep3B cells with or without IFN-α (1 000 U/ml). On day 14, PBMC were harvested and subjected to cytolytic assay. The ^{51}Cr release assay was employed to test the cytolytic activity of stimulated cells. Target cells (parental

Hep3B) were labeled with ^{51}Cr and incubated with effector cells at various effector/target (E/T) ratios. Supernatants were obtained after incubation and subjected to γ-counting. To analyze HLA restriction in cytotoxicity, anti-HLA-ABC monoclonal antibody and anti-HLA DR monoclonal antibody were added at the beginning of the assay.

Tumor Growth of Murine B7-1-Transfected HCC Cells in Mice

To establish HCC cells strongly expressing B7-1, BNL cells were transfected with BCMGS-murine B7-1 expression vector. B7-1 expression was evaluated by flow cytometry. After 1×10^6 cells of BNL cells or murine B7-1-transfected BNL cells (BNL-mB7-1) were injected subcutaneously into the back of each syngeneic BALB/c mouse, the mice were observed for subcutaneous tumor formation.

Immunization of Mice

Each BALB/c mouse was immunized intraperitoneally with 1×10^6 mitomycin-C-treated BNL-mB7-1 cells four times at 0, 1, 2, and 3 weeks before subcutaneous injection of BNL cells into the back of syngeneic BALB/c mice. Control mice were immunized with phosphate-buffered saline (PBS) intraperitoneally. Immediately after the final vaccination, 1×10^6 BNL cells were injected subcutaneously into the back of both immunized and control BALB/c mice.

Cytolytic Assay

Cytolytic assays were performed approximately 2 weeks after the final immunization. The spleen cells from immunized mice were cocultured with mitomycin-C-treated BNL-mB7-1 cells. After 7 days of incubation, cytotoxic effector lymphocytes were subjected to cytolytic assay. The ^{51}Cr release assay was employed to test the cytolytic activity of stimulated cells.

Results

Expression of B7-1, B7-2, and HLA Class I on Human HCC Cells

The expression of B7-1, B7-2, and HLA class I was studied by flow cytometry. As shown in Fig. 1, HepG2 cells expressed B7-1 and B7-2 molecules on the cell surface with a low positive cell rate and expressed HLA class I with a high positive cell rate. The results of flow cytometric analysis of seven HCC cell lines are summarized in Table 1. All human HCC cell lines expressed B7-1, B7-2, and HLA class I on their cell surface. However, the positive cell rates of B7-1 and B7-2 on all HCC cell lines were less than 9%. On the other hand, in five of the seven HCC cell lines, the positive cell rates of HLA class I antigen were more than 97% and Huh-6 and HB611 showed about 32% positive cell rates (Table 1).

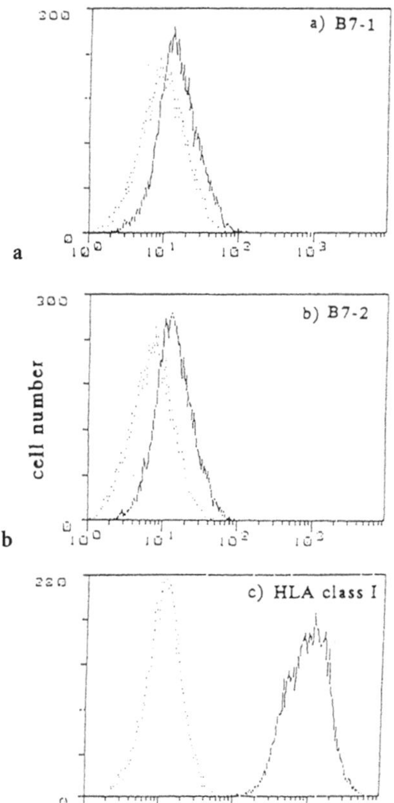

Fig. 1a–c. Flow cytometric analysis of B7-1, B7-2, and human leukocyte antigen (HLA) class I expressions on HepG2 cells. **a** The profile of B7-1-stained cells (*solid line*) is superimposed on the profile of staining with the isotype control (*dotted line*). **b** The profile of B7-2-stained cells (*solid line*) is superimposed on the profile of staining with the isotype control (*dotted line*). **c** The profile of HLA class I-stained cells (*solid line*) is superimposed on the profile of staining with the isotype control (*dotted line*)

Table 1. Expression of B7-1, B7-2, and human leukocyte antigen (HLA) class I on human hepatocellular carcinoma (HCC) cell lines

	Positive cell (%)						
	Hep3B	HepG2	KYN-3	PLC/PRF/5	Huh-7	Huh-6	HB611
B7-1	1.7	6.9	3.2	5.1	2.7	6.3	9.0
	(8.8)	(18.8)	(26.9)	(16.0)	(25.6)	(43.3)	(43.7)
B7-2	3.2	8.6	3.5	7.7	7.0	4.3	7.1
	(19.0)	(48.2)	(5.9)	(18.1)	(29.9)	(32.0)	(42.9)
HLA class I	99.9	99.9	98.8	99.9	97.7	32.6	32.3
	(2004.7)	(1185.9)	(5587.1)	(4031.6)	(1202.3)	(237.7)	(385.2)

Mean fluorescence intensity of stained HCC cells is given in parentheses.

Induction of B7-1 and B7-2 Expression by Cytokine

We investigated cytokine regulation of B7-1 and B7-2 expression on human HCC cell lines. The upregulation of B7-1 expression after treatment with IFN-α (1 000 U/ml) was observed in six HCC cell lines, and upregulation after treatment with IFN-γ (1 000 U/ml) was observed in six HCC cell lines. IL-12 (10 ng/ml) showed no effect on the expression of B7-1 in all HCC cell lines (Table 2). On the other hand, the upregulation of B7-2 expression after treatment with IFN-α (1 000 U/ml) was observed in four HCC cell lines and upregulation after treatment with IFN-γ (1 000 U/ml) was observed in four HCC cell lines. IL-12 (10 ng/ml) showed no effect on B7-2 expression in any of the HCC cell lines (Table 3).

Role of B7-1 in the Induction of Primary Cytolytic Activity Against Human HCC

To investigate the amount of expression inducing effective antitumor immunity, we examined the cytolytic activity against parental Hep3B cells generated by B7-1-transfected, cytokine-treated, or untreated Hep3B cells. As shown in Fig. 2a, B7-1-transfected Hep3B cells elicited primary cytolytic activity against parental Hep3B cells, but IFN-α-treated Hep3B cells and parental Hep3B cells could not. These results

Table 2. Induction of B7-1 on human hepatocellular carcinoma (HCC) cells by cytokines

Cell line	Stimulation index		
	IFN-α (1 000 U/ml)	IFN-γ (1 000 U/ml)	IL-12 (10 ng/ml)
Hep3B	1.72 (15.2)	2.48 (21.9)	1.18 (10.4)
HepG2	1.26 (23.7)	1.58 (29.8)	1.19 (22.4)
KYN-3	1.53 (41.3)	1.81 (48.7)	1.18 (31.8)
PLC/PRF/5	3.48 (55.6)	1.32 (21.1)	1.08 (17.4)
Huh-7	1.49 (38.2)	1.26 (32.2)	1.28 (33.0)
Huh-6	1.45 (62.8)	3.50 (151.4)	1.20 (51.9)
HB611	1.55 (67.7)	1.55 (67.8)	1.19 (51.9)

IFN, interferon; IL, interleukin. Mean fluorescence intensity of stained HCC cells in parentheses.

Table 3. Induction of B7-2 on human HCC cells by cytokines

Cell line	Stimulation index		
	IFN-α (1 000 U/ml)	IFN-γ (1 000 U/ml)	IL-12 (10 ng/ml)
Hep3B	2.10 (39.9)	1.58 (30.0)	1.02 (19.4)
HepG2	1.11 (53.3)	1.52 (73.4)	1.02 (49.4)
KYN-3	1.53 (9.0)	1.76 (10.4)	0.98 (5.8)
PLC/PRF/5	1.62 (29.3)	1.53 (27.7)	1.02 (18.4)
Huh-7	2.06 (61.6)	1.09 (32.6)	1.16 (34.8)
Huh-6	1.34 (42.8)	1.27 (40.7)	1.18 (37.8)
HB611	1.39 (59.6)	1.13 (48.5)	1.00 (42.9)

Mean fluorescence intensity of stained HCC cells in parentheses.

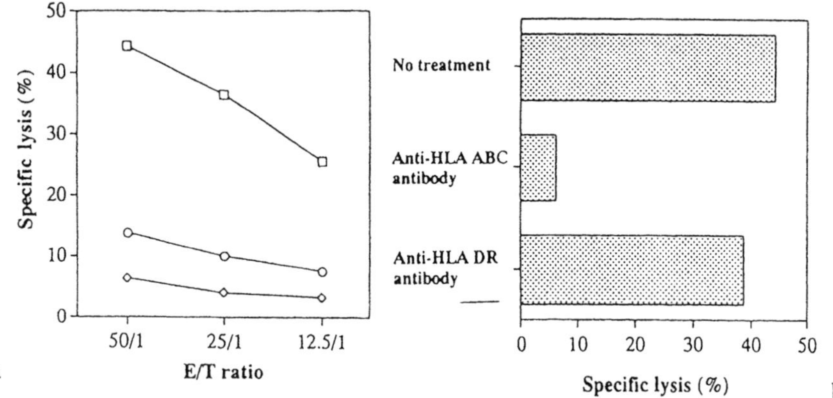

Fig. 2. a Induction of primary cytolytic activity in mixed lymphocytes and tumor cultures (MLTC) by B7-1-transfected Hep3B cells, cytokine-treated Hep3B cells, or untreated Hep3B cells from normal volunteers. Similar results were obtained in two experiments. *Squares*, B7-1-transfected Hep3B cells; *circles*, interferon-α-treated Hep3B cells; *diamonds*, untreated Hep3B cells. **b** Changes in cytolytic activity caused by anti-HLA antibody treatments in a HLA partially matched volunteer. Effector/target (E/T) ratio was 50:1. Representative results are shown. *No treatment*, cytolytic activity induced by B7-1-transfected Hep3B cells in ^{51}Cr release assay; *anti-HLA ABC antibody*, cytolytic activity induced by B7-1-transfected Hep3B cells when anti-HLA ABC antibody was added in ^{51}Cr release assay; *anti-HLA DR antibody*, cytolytic activity induced by B7-1-transfected Hep3B cells when anti-HLA DR antibody was added in ^{51}Cr release assay

demonstrated that HCC cells with strong B7-1 expression could stimulate human lymphocytes to show cytolytic activity against parental HCC cells but HCC cells with weak B7-1 expression could not. Cytolytic activity was decreased with anti-HLA ABC antibody but not with anti-HLA DR antibody (Fig. 2b).

Tumor Growth of B7-1-Transfected Mouse HCC Cells in Syngeneic Animals

We examined the tumor growth of BNL-mB7-1 and BNL in syngeneic BALB/c mice to determine whether increased B7-1 expression would have any effect on the growth of mouse HCC cells in vivo. In BALB/c mice, the tumor growth of BNL-mB7-1 cells was significantly inhibited compared with that of the parental BNL cells (Fig. 3).

Immunization with B7-1 Transfectant

To examine the ability of BNL-mB7-1 cells to induce a protective effect against parental BNL tumors, we tried to vaccinate mice with B7-1-transfected HCC cells. The tumor growth of parental BNL cells after vaccination with BNL-mB7-1 cells was significantly inhibited compared with that with PBS (Fig. 4).

Cytolytic Activity Against Mouse HCC Cells

We investigated whether cytolytic activity against parental BNL cells was generated by immunization with B7-1-transfected BNL cells. Splenocytes from mice immunized

Fig. 3. Growth rate of tumors developing after subcutaneous inoculation of 1×10^6 cells of parental BNL 1ME A.7R.1 or mouse B7-1-transfected BNL 1ME A.7R.1 in syngeneic BALB/c mouse. *Diamonds*, parental BNL 1ME A.7R.1 HCC cells ($n = 10$); *Squares*, B7-1-transfected BNL 1ME A.7R.1 HCC cells ($n = 10$). Each data point represents the mean ± SE

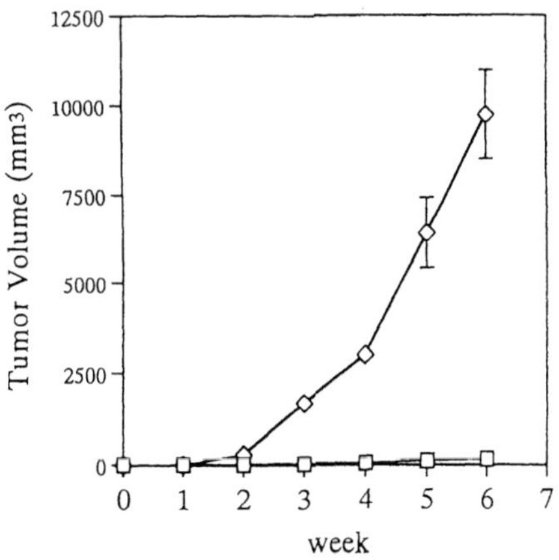

Fig. 4 Effect of vaccination with B7-1-transfected BNL 1ME A.7R.1 Hepatocellular carcinoma (HCC) cells on tumor growth of parental BNL 1ME A.7R.1 HCC cells. BALB/c mice were immunized intraperitoneally with either 1×10^6 of mitomycin-C-treated BNL-mB7-1 cells or PBS three times. *Diamonds*, control vaccination ($n = 10$); *Squares*, B7-1-transfected BNL 1ME A.7R.1 HCC cells vaccination ($n = 10$). Each data point represents the mean ± SE

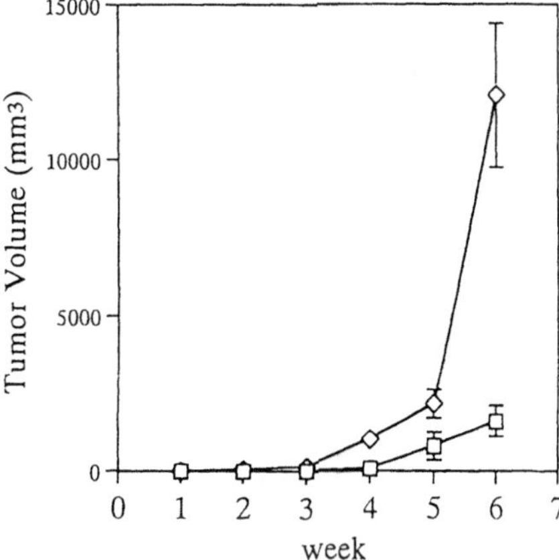

with BNL-mB7-1 cells showed cytolytic activity against parental BNL cells, but those from mice immunized with PBS showed minimal cytolytic activity (Fig. 5). These results demonstrated that immunization with BNL-mB7-1 could induce cytolytic activity against parental BNL cells in vivo.

Discussion

The present flow cytometric studies using monoclonal antibodies against B7-1 and B7-2 showed that HCC cells express costimulatory molecules B7-1 and B7-2 on their cell surface with low positive cell rates. On the other hand, HLA class I is strongly expressed on human HCC cells. These results suggest that low expression of B7-1 and B7-2 on the majority of the HCC cells causes the inability of tumor antigens to stimulate an effective immune response, which may induce an anergic state in T cells. Taken together with these findings, our results seemed to suggest that antitumor

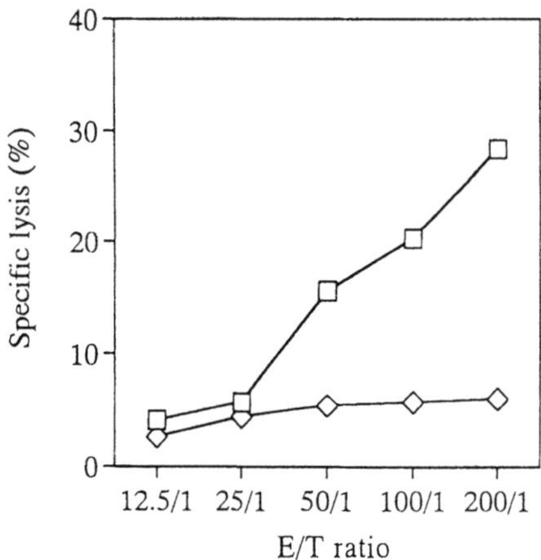

Fig. 5 Cytolytic activity of spleen cells derived from mice immunized with mitomycin-C-treated BNL-mB7-1 cells. The spleen cells from immunized mice were taken 2 weeks after the final injection and were cocultured in vitro with BNL-mB7-1 cells. *Squares*, cytolytic activity immunized with B7-1-transfected BNL 1ME A.7R.1 HCC cells; *diamonds*, cytolytic activity of control vaccination

immunity against human HCC could be induced if the expression levels of these costimulatory molecules were higher.

There have been several reports on antitumor immunotherapy by inducing B7-1 or B7-2 expression on tumor cells to stimulate more effective antitumor immune responses [17–23]. When the B7-1 or B7-2 gene is transduced and expressed in tumor cells, it renders them susceptible to T-cell-mediated rejection, and sometimes curative immunity against wild-type tumors can be induced in murine tumor models. Mixed lymphocytes and tumor cultures demonstrated that B7-1-transfected Hep3B cells could induce primary cytolytic activity against Hep3B cells but that cytokine-treated and untreated Hep3B cells could not. These findings illustrated that strong expression of B7-1 on HCC cells plays a crucial role in the induction of primary cytolytic activity in vitro but that minimal increase of B7-1 following cytokine treatments does not. Our findings raise the possibility that human HCC cells, made to strongly express B7-1 by ex vivo or in vivo transfection, could be used to induce antitumor immunity against human HCC.

In our tumor growth study, B7-1-transfected HCC cells were significantly inhibited compared with parental HCC cells when implanted into syngeneic BALB/c mice. These results suggested that strong expression of B7-1 molecules on HCC cells can increase the immunogenicity of mouse HCC cells in vivo. Chen et al. reported that rejection of immunogenic tumor, but not the rejection of poorly immunogenic tumor, could be induced by B7-1 expression [27]. On the other hand, Coughlin et al. reported that strong expression of B7-1 on tumor cells could delay tumor development and prolong duration of survival with tumor in the poorly immunogenic tumor model [28]. In the present study, strong expression of B7-1 on HCC cells could not induce complete rejection of implanted B7-1-transfected HCC cells but could delay tumor development. These results are consistent with the observation of Coughlin et al. and confirmed that the strong expression of B7-1 molecules on tumor cells is useful for inducting an antitumor effect against poorly immunogenic tumors.

In this study, we investigated whether immunization with B7-1-gene-transfected HCC cells can induce systemic tumor immunity and inhibit the growth of parental HCC cells. We found that tumor growth of parental HCC cells was significantly inhibited, with delay of tumor development. Furthermore, our lymphocyte findings demonstrated that splenocytes from mice immunized with B7-1-transfected HCC cells showed cytolytic activity against parental BNL cells, while those from splenocytes from control mice only showed minimal cytolytic activity. These results raise the possibility that immunization of B7-1-transfected human HCC cells obtained from tumor biopsy or surgical resection may offer the benefit of suppressing HCC recurrence and prolonging patient life.

In conclusion, costimulatory molecules (B7-1 and B7-2) are expressed on the human HCC cell surface but at much lower levels than HLA class I. Primary cytolytic activity against HCC cells was effectively generated by B7-1-transfected HCC cells in vitro. The tumor growth of B7-1-transfected HCC cells can be significantly inhibited in syngeneic mice, and vaccination with B7-1-transfected HCC cells can induce anti-tumor immunity against parental HCC cells. We speculate that vaccination with B7-1-gene-transfected tumor cells may be useful in immunogene therapy against poorly immunogenic HCC.

References

1. Schwartz RH (1992) Costimulation of T lymphocytes, the role of CD28, CTLA-4, and B7/BB1 in interleukin-2 production and immunotherapy. Cell 71:1065–1079
2. Liu Y, Linsley PS (1992) Costimulation of T cell growth. Curr Opin Immunol 4:265–270
3. Allison JP (1994) CD28-B7 interaction in T cell activation. Curr Opin Immunol 6:414–419
4. Linsley PS, Ledbetter JA (1993) The role of the CD28 receptor during T-cell responses to antigen. Annu Rev Immunol 11:191–212
5. Gimmi CD, Freeman GJ, Gribben JG, Gray G, Nadler LM (1993) Human T-cell clonal anergy is induced by antigen presentation in the absence of B7 costimulation. Proc Natl Acad Sci USA 90:6586–6590
6. Harding FA, McArthur JG, Gross JA, Raulet DH, Allison JP (1992) CD28-mediated signaling co-stimulates murine T cells and prevents induction of anergy in T-cell clones. Nature (Lond) 356:607–609
7. Linsley PS, Clark EA, Ledbetter JA (1990) T-cell activation antigen CD28 mediates adhesion with B cells by interacting with activation antigen B7/BB1. Proc Natl Acad Sci USA 87:5031–5035
8. Linsley PS, Brady W, Grosmaire L, Aruffo A, Damle NK, Ledbetter JA (1990) Binding of the B cell activation antigen B7 to CD28 costimulates T cell proliferation and interleukin-2 mRNA accumulation. J Exp Med 173:721–730
9. Linsley PS, Brady W, Urnes M, Grosmaire L, Damle NK, Ledbetter JA (1991) CTLA-4 is a second receptor for the B cell activation antigen B7. J Exp Med 174:561–569
10. Freeman GJ, Freedman AS, Segil JM, Lee G, Whitman JF, Nadler LM (1989) B7, a new member of the Ig superfamily with unique expression on activated and neoplastic B cells. J Immunol 143:2714–2722
11. June CH, Bluestone JA, Nadler LM, Thompson CB (1994) The B7 and CD28 receptor families. Immunol Today 15:321–331
12. Azuma M, Ito D, Yagita H, Okumura K, Phillips JH, Lanier LL, Somoza C (1993) B70 antigen is a second ligand for CTLA-4 and CD28. Nature (Lond) 366:76–79

13. Freeman GJ, Gribben JG, Boussiotis VA, Ng JW, Restivo VA, Lombard LA, Gray GS, Nadler LM (1993) Cloning of B7-2: a CTLA-4 counter-receptor that costimulates human T cell proliferation. Science 262:909–911

14. Freeman GJ, Borriello F, Hodes RJ, Reiser H, Gribben JG, Ng JW, Kim J, Goldberg JM, Hathcok K, Laszlo G, Lombard LA, Wang S, Gray GS, Nadler LM, Sharpe AH (1993) Murine B7-2, an alternative CTLA-4 counter-receptor that costimulates T cell proliferation and interleukin 2 production. J Exp Med 178:2185–2192

15. Chen C, Gault A, Shen LJ, Nabavi N (1994) Molecular cloning and expression of T cell costimulatory molecule ETC-1 and its characterization as B7-2. J Immunol 152:4929–4936

16. Yokochi T, Holley RD, Clark EA (1982) B lymphocyte antigen (BB1) expressed on Epstein-Barr virus-activated B cell blasts, B lymphoblastoid cell lines, and Burkitt's lymphomas. J Immunol 128:823–827

17. Chen L, Linsley PS, Helstrom KE (1993) Costimulation of T cells for tumor immunity. Immunol Today 14:483–486

18. Chen L, Ashe S, Brady WA, Hellstrom I, Hellstrom KE, Ledbetter JA, McGowan P, Linsley PS (1992) Costimulation of antitumor immunity by the B7 counter-receptor for the T lymphocyte molecules CD28 and CTLA-4. Cell 71:1093–1102

19. Townsend SE, Allison JP (1993) Tumor rejection after direct costimulation of CD8$^+$ T cells by B7-transfected melanoma cells. Science 259:368–370

20. Baskar S, Ostrand-Rosenberg S, Nabavi N, Nadler LM, Freemana GJ, Glimcher LH (1993) Constitutive expression of B7 restores immunogenicity of tumor cells expressing truncated MHC class II molecules. Proc Natl Acad Sci USA 90:5687–5690

21. Ramarathinam L, Castle M, Wu Y, Liu Y (1994) T cell costimulation by B7/BB1 induces CD8 T-cell-dependent tumor rejection: an important role of B7/BB1 in the induction, recruitment, and effector function of antitumor T cells. J Exp Med 179:1205–1214

22. Li Y, McGowan P, Hellstrom I, Hellstrom KE, Chen L (1994) Costimulation of tumor-reactive CD4$^+$ and CD8$^+$ T lymphocytes by B7, a natural ligand for CD28, can be used to treat established mouse melanoma. J Immunol 153;421–428

23. Yang G, Hellstrom KE, Hellstrom I, Chen L (1995) Antitumor immunity elicited by tumor cells transfected with B7-2, a second ligand for CD28/CTLA-4 costimulatory molecules. J Immunol 154:2794–2800

24. Paroli M, Carloni G, Franco A, De-Petrillo G, Alfani E, Perrone A, Barnaba V (1994) Human hepatoma cells expressing MHC antigens display accessory cell function dependence on LFA1/ICAM-1 interaction. Immunology 82(2):215–221

25. Momosaki S, Yano H, Ogasawara S, Higaki K, Hisaka T, Kojiro M (1995) Expression of intercellular adhesion molecule 1 in human hepatocellular carcinoma. Hepatology 22:1708–1713

26. Tatsumi T, Takehara T, Katayama K, Mochizuki K, Yamamoto M, Kanto T, Sasaki Y, Kasahara A, Hayashi N (1997) Expression of costimulatory molecules B7-1 (CD80) and B7-2 (CD86) on human hepatocellular carcinoma. Hepatology 25:1108–1114

27. Chen L, McGowan P, Ashe S, Johnston J, Li Y, Hellstrom I, Hellstrom KE (1994) Tumor immunogenicity determines the effect of B7 costimulation on T cell-mediated tumor immunity, J Exp Med 179:523–532

28. Coughlin CM, Wysocka M, Kurzawa HL, Lee WMF, Trinchieri G, Eck SL (1995) B7-1 and interleukin-12 synergistically induce effective antitumor immunity. Cancer Res 55:4980–4987

Clonal Deletion, A Novel Strategy of Cancer Control that Falls Between Cancer Chemoprevention and Cancer Chemotherapy: A Clinical Experience in Liver Cancer

HISATAKA MORIWAKI, MASATAKA OKUNO, YOSHIMUNE SHIRATORI, ICHIRO YASUDA, and YASUTOSHI MUTO

Summary. Liver cancer is characterized by multistep and multicentric carcinogenesis. The liver of patients with chronic liver disease essentially contains multiple preneoplastic or latent malignant clones of liver cancer. Current strategies against liver carcinogenesis contain a pitfall because the premalignant and latent malignant clones that have accumulated gene mutations are left without any specific therapies. Once a novel therapeutic strategy is established targeting such preneoplastic or latent malignant clones, large beneficial effects are subsequently anticipated. A randomized controlled clinical study demonstrated that the administration of acyclic retinoid significantly reduced the incidence of second primary liver cancers in patients who had undergone curative removal of their preceding liver cancers. The clones that secrete the lectin-reactive fraction of α-fetoprotein (AFP-L3) have been deleted as well as inhibited by acyclic retinoid in the patients' remnant liver. Such clonal deletion of AFP-L3-secreting cells may well contribute to the reduction of second primary liver cancers. Two possible pathways for clonal deletion can be proposed, including induction of immediate apoptosis and differentiation induction followed by the recovery of programmed cell death. Our experience in liver cancer is the first that demonstrated clinically the deletion of preneoplastic or latent malignant clones. Supposing that every cancer takes the course of multistep carcinogenesis and essentially has a preneoplastic or latent malignant clone before clinical detection, clonal deletion therapy will have a large share in a general anticancer strategy in the near future.

Key words. Hepatocellular carcinoma, Cancer chemoprevention, Retinoid, Differentiation induction, Clonal deletion, Alpha-fetoprotein, Apoptosis

Introduction

The development of malignancies including liver cancer takes the course of multistep carcinogenesis (Fig. 1). In addition, liver cancer is also characterized by multicentric carcinogenesis. The latter is understood by a concept of "field cancerization" [1], that

First Department of Internal Medicine, Gifu University School of Medicine, 40 Tsukasa-machi, Gifu 500-8705, Japan

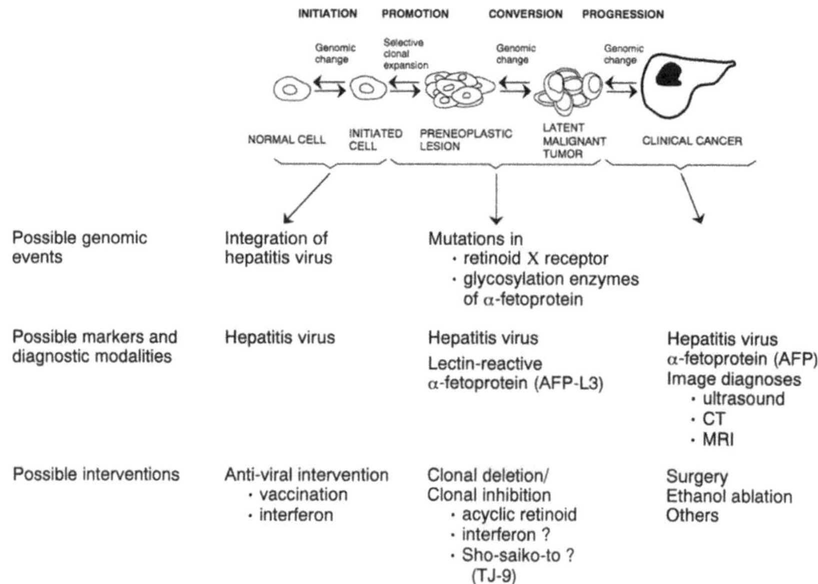

Fig. 1. Schematic illustration of multistep carcinogenesis of the liver. Preneoplastic or latent malignant clones that have mutations in retinoid X receptor (RXR) and in glycosylation enzymes of α-fetoprotein are possible targets of the clonal deletion therapy of liver cancer by acyclic retinoid

an organ or a tissue, the liver, for example, is exposed as a whole field to a continuous carcinogenic insult such as hepatitis virus infection or alcohol drinking. The liver subsequently develops multiple independent clones that have damaged and mutated DNA. Hence, it is supposed that a number of lines of multistep carcinogenesis are progressing in parallel in the liver of hepatitis virus carriers or of alcoholics. In other words, the liver of patients with chronic liver disease essentially contains multiple preneoplastic or latent malignant clones of liver cancer.

Current Strategies and Their Pitfalls

As current strategies against liver carcinogenesis, prevention of hepatitis virus infection using γ-globulin and vaccination [2] and the removal of infected hepatitis viruses by interferon have been established. For clinically detectable liver cancers, surgical resection, ethanol ablation, chemotherapy, radiation, and other therapeutic modalities are available. However, as illustrated in Fig. 1, these approaches cover only both ends of multistep carcinogenesis. A large intermediate portion, that is, patients with chronic liver disease who have mutated clones in their liver, are left without any specific therapies against their premalignant or latent malignant clones.

Proposal of "Clonal Deletion"

Once a novel therapeutic strategy is established targeting such preneoplastic or latent malignant clones, large beneficial effects are subsequently anticipated. As direct effects, first, the number of hepatoma patients who require intensive therapy will be markedly reduced and, second, the development of second primary hepatomas will be inhibited in patients who already have received treatment for their initial hepatomas. These two effects will bring an improvement in cost-effectiveness in the medical care of patients with chronic liver disease by eliminating costly therapies directed at liver cancer. Actually, death from liver cancer accounts for approximately 27000 persons per year in Japan [3] and, when clonal deletion therapy becomes effective, the direct as well as indirect costs for the care of patients with liver cancer will no longer be required. In addition, an elevation in cost benefit as a socioeconomic measure will be also achieved by improving the quality of life and long-term survival of the cirrhotic patients because the 5-year survival rate has not yet reached 50% in those patients once they develop liver cancer [4].

Clinical Experience

In a randomized controlled study, we demonstrated that the administration of acyclic retinoid, an open-chain C-20 analog [5,6], significantly reduced the incidence of second primary liver cancers in patients who had undergone curative removal of their preceding liver cancers [7]. In this study, we observed that the serum level of a particular isoform of α-fetoprotein (AFP), a lectin-reactive fraction of AFP (AFP-L3), was significantly decreased after 12 months of treatment with acyclic retinoid (at entry: median, 0 ng/ml, range, 0–8.4 ng/ml; after 12 months: median, 0 ng/ml, range, 0–0.13 ng/ml; $P < .05$ by the paired t-test for 21 patients) [8]. This reduction was brought about by the deletion of AFP-L3 in patients who were positive at entry (Fig. 2). Because spontaneous disappearance of AFP-L3 was not observed in the placebo group, we concluded that acyclic retinoid deleted premalignant or latent malignant clones that produced and secreted AFP-L3 [8]. In addition, the number of AFP-L3-positive patients in the placebo group significantly increased after 12 months ($P < .05$) (Fig. 2) [8]. Because there was no patient in whom AFP-L3 newly appeared in the acyclic retinoid group, it was suggested that the development of AFP-L3-producing clones was also inhibited by the agent [8]. As other isoforms of or total concentrations of AFP were not affected by acyclic retinoid, its effects are likely specific on the clones that secrete AFP-L3.

In the follow-up period after 12 months of drug administration, AFP-L3-positive patients developed second primary liver cancers at a significantly higher rate than AFP-L3-negative patients did ($P = .03$) [8]. Serum AFP-L3 predicts the presence of premalignant or malignant clones in the cirrhotic liver [9–11]. Our clinical observation strongly suggests that clones that secrete AFP-L3 have been deleted as well as inhibited by acyclic retinoid in the patients' remnant liver. Such clonal deletion of AFP-L3-secreting cells may well contribute to the reduction of second primary liver cancers.

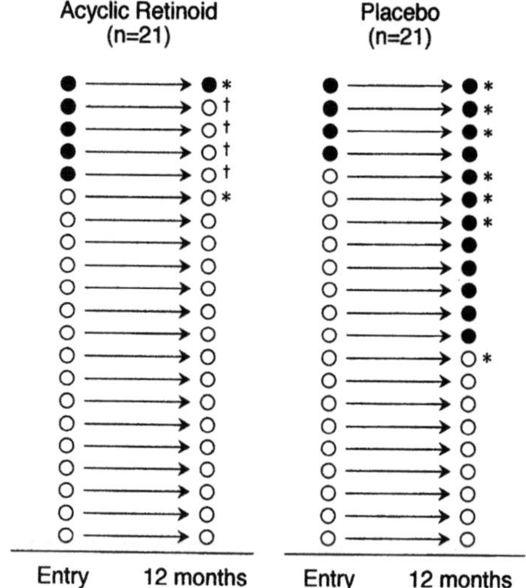

Fig. 2. Successful clonal deletion therapy of second primary liver cancer. Patients indicated by *closed circles* have preneoplastic or latent malignant clones that secrete lectin-reactive α-fetoprotein (AFP-L3); patients indicated by *open circles* do not have such clones. Acyclic retinoid or placebo was administered for 12 months to each of 21 randomized patients (see [7,8]), and serum AFP-L3 was determined at entry and after 12 months. †, Patients in whom AFP-L3-producing clones have been deleted by acyclic retinoid. Incidence of AFP-L3-positive patients after 12 months was significantly lower in the acyclic retinoid group (1 in 21) than in the placebo group (12 in 21) ($P < .001$), while that at entry was not different significantly between the two groups (5 in 21 and 4 in 21, respectively). *, Patients who subsequently developed second primary liver cancers

Theory and Mechanisms

Successful clonal deletion therapy requires the removal of the clone. Two possible pathways can be proposed including induction of immediate apoptosis and differentiation induction followed by the recovery of programmed cell death [6]. The latter mechanism has been recently defined as slow apoptosis [12]. As to liver cancer, we demonstrated that acyclic retinoid induced apoptosis in cultures of human hepatoma-derived cell lines within several hours without inducing cell differentiation [13]. This immediate apoptosis was brought by interrupting the autocrine–paracrine growth stimulation by down-regulating the expression of both transforming growth factor-α (TGF-α) and its receptor, epidermal growth factor receptor (EGFR) [14].

The second mechanism is a differentiation induction characterized by the recovery of albumin gene expression and downregulation of AFP mRNA [15]. This differentiation induction may be mediated by the binding of acyclic retinoid with its receptor, retinoid X receptor (RXR) [15].

In the process of liver carcinogenesis, possible mutations are suggested to be introduced in the RXR gene [16]. These mutations may impair the physiological processing of RXR protein and the subsequent signal transduction [17]. An abnormality in another retinoid receptor, retinoic acid receptor (RAR), is also associated with the development of a hematological malignancy, acute promyelocytic leukemia, by the dominant-negative inhibition of the physiological signal-transducing pathway of cell differentiation [18]. Administration of a pharmacological amount of the receptor ligand, all-*trans* retinoic acid, recovers differentiation and apoptosis of the leukemia cells [19]. Thus, in cases both of liver cancer and of acute promyelocytic leukemia, recovery of the signal transduction via nuclear retinoid receptors by retinoid therapy [20,21] can be regarded as a gene-targeting therapy of carcinogenesis. In this aspect, acute promyelocytic leukemia and at least some liver cancer can be recognized as genomic nuclear receptor diseases (16,21–23).

Two other studies have shown inhibition of the development of liver cancer in cirrhotic patients using Sho-saiko-to [24] and interferon-α [25]. The clonal deletion mechanism might have also worked in addition to their antiinflammatory action and antiviral action.

Future Direction

Clonal deletion was proposed previously as a step in cancer chemoprevention strategy by Hong and Lotan [26–28] but has never been demonstrated even in successful clinical prevention trials [29,30]. Our experience in liver cancer [8] is the first to demonstrate clinically the deletion of preneoplastic or latent malignant clones. Moreover, basic research suggests that clonal deletion is a therapy rather than a method of prevention, targeting a particular clone that has specific gene mutation(s) such as in the RXR gene and the glycosylation enzymes of AFP. Even when the target clones at the latent stage cannot be detected by image diagnoses, serum markers such as AFP-L3 can indicate their presence. Supposing that every cancer takes the course of multistep carcinogenesis and essentially has a preneoplastic or latent malignant clone before clinical detection, clonal deletion therapy will have a large share in a general anticancer strategy, as proposed against lung cancer, for example [31], in the near future. An extensive effort should also be made to identify a reliable marker, either genomic, serum, or histological, to indicate the presence of such target clones in other cancers.

Acknowledgment. The authors thank Dr. Hirota Fujiki, Director, Saitama Cancer Center Research Institute, for his valuable discussions. This work was supported in part by grants-in-aid from the Ministry of Education, Science, Sports and Culture (H.M., M.O.) and from the Ministry of Health and Welfare of Japan (H.M.).

References

1. Slaughter PD, Southwick HW, Smejkel W (1953) "Field cancerization" in oral stratified epithelium: clinical implications of multicentric cancer. Cancer (Phila) 6:963–968
2. Chang M-H, Chen C-J, Lai M-S, Hsu H-M, Wu T-C, Kong M-S, Liang D-C, Shau W-Y, Chen D-S (1997) Universal hepatitis B vaccination in Taiwan and the incidence of hepatocellular carcinoma in children. N Engl J Med 336:1855–1859

3. Health and Welfare Statistics Association (1996) Annual report of disease-related deaths in Japan. J Health Welfare Stat 43(suppl 9):47–59
4. Liver Cancer Study Group of Japan (1997) Survey and follow-up study of primary liver cancer in Japan. Acta Hepatol Jpn 38:317–330
5. Muto Y, Moriwaki H (1984) Antitumor activities of vitamin A and its derivatives. J Natl Cancer Inst 73:1389–1393
6. Muto Y, Moriwaki H (1991) Acyclic retinoids and cancer chemoprevention. Pure Appl Chem 63:157–160
7. Muto Y, Moriwaki H, Ninomiya M, Adachi S, Saito A, Takasaki KT, Tanaka T, Tsurumi K, Okuno M, Tomita E, Nakamura T, Kojima T (1996) Prevention of second primary tumors by an acyclic retinoid, polyprenoic acid, in patients with hepatocellular carcinoma. N Engl J Med 334:1561–1567
8. Moriwaki H, Yasuda I, Shiratori Y, Uematsu T, Okuno M, Muto Y (1997) Deletion of serum lectin-reactive α-fetoprotein by acyclic retinoid: a potent biomarker in the chemoprevention of second primary hepatoma. Clin Cancer Res 3:727–731
9. Sato Y, Nakata K, Kato Y, Shima M, Ishii N, Koji T, Taketa K, Nagataki S (1993) Early recognition of hepatocellular carcinoma based on altered profiles of alpha-fetoprotein. N Engl J Med 328:1802–1806
10. Shiraki K, Takase K, Tameda Y, Hamada M, Kosaka Y, Nakano T (1995) A clinical study of lectin-reactive alpha-fetoprotein as an early indicator of hepatocellular carcinoma in the follow-up of cirrhotic patients. Hepatology 22:802–807
11. Yamashita F, Tanaka M, Satomura S, Tanikawa K (1996) Prognostic significance of lens culinaris agglutinin A-reactive α-fetoprotein in small hepatocellular carcinomas. Gastroenterology 111:996–1001
12. Au JL-S, Li D, Gan Y, Gao X, Johnson AL, Johnston J, Millenbaugh NJ, Jang SH, Kuh H-J, Chen C-T, Wientjes G (1998) Pharmacodynamics of immediate and delayed effects of paclitaxel: role of slow apoptosis and intracellular drug retention. Cancer Res 58:2141–2148
13. Nakamura N, Shidoji Y, Yamada Y, Hatakeyama H, Moriwaki H, Muto Y (1995) Induction of apoptosis by acyclic retinoid in the human hepatoma-derived cell line, HuH-7. Biochem Biophys Res Commun 207:382–388
14. Nakamura N, Shidoji Y, Moriwaki H, Muto Y (1996) Apoptosis in human hepatoma cell line by 4,5-didehydro geranylgeranoic acid (acyclic retinoid) via down-regulation of transforming growth factor-α. Biochem Biophys Res Commun 219:100–104
15. Yamada Y, Shidoji Y, Fukutomi Y, Ishikawa T, Kaneko T, Nakagama H, Imawari M, Moriwaki H, Muto Y (1994) Positive and negative regulations of albumin gene expression by retinoids in human hepatoma cell lines. Mol Carcinog 10:151–158
16. Matsushima-Nishiwaki R, Shidoji Y, Nishiwaki S, Moriwaki H, Muto Y (1996) Limited degradation of retinoid X receptor by calpain. Biochem Biophys Res Commun 225:946–951
17. Matsushima-Nishiwaki R, Shidoji Y, Moriwaki H, Muto Y (1996) Aberrant metabolism of retinoid X receptor proteins in human hepatocellular carcinoma. Mol Cell Endocrinol 121:179–190
18. de The H, Lavau C, Marchio A, Chomienne C, Degos L, Dejean A (1991) The PML-RAR alpha fusion mRNA generated by the t(15:17) translocation in acute promyelocytic leukemia encodes a functionally altered RAR. Cell 66:675–684
19. Huang ME, Yu-Chen Y, Shu-Rong C, Lu MX, Zhao L, Gu LJ, Wang ZY (1988) Use of all-*trans* retinoic acid in the treatment of acute promyelocytic leukemia. Blood 72:567–572
20. Araki H, Shidoji Y, Yamada Y, Moriwaki H, Muto Y (1995) Retinoid agonist activities of synthetic geranyl geranoic acid derivatives. Biochem Biophys Res Commun 209:66–72

21. Chomienne C, Fenaux P, Degos L (1996) Retinoid differentiation therapy in promyelocytic leukemia. FASEB J 10:1025–1030
22. de The H (1996) Altered retinoic acid receptors. FASEB J 10:955–960
23. Dejean A, Bougueleret L, Crzeschick K, Tiollais P (1986) Hepatitis virus DNA integration in a sequence homologous to v-erbA and steroid receptors genes in a hepatocellular carcinoma. Nature (Lond) 322:70–72
24. Oka H, Yamamoto S, Kuroki T, Harihara S, Marumo T, Kim SR, Monna T, Kobayashi K, Tango T (1995) Prospective study of chemoprevention of hepatocellular carcinoma with Sho-saiko-to (TJ-9). Cancer (Phila) 76:743–749
25. Nishiguchi S, Kuroki T, Nakatani S, Morimoto H, Taketa T, Nakajima S, Shimi S, Seki S, Kobayashi K, Otani S (1995) Randomized trial of effects of interferon-α on the incidence of hepatocellular carcinoma in chronic active hepatitis C with cirrhosis. Lancet 346:1051–1055
26. Hong WK, Lippman SM, Hittelman WN, Lotan R (1995) Retinoid chemoprevention of aerodigestive cancer: from basic research to the clinic. Clin Cancer Res 1:677–686
27. Lotan R (1996) Retinoids in cancer chemoprevention. FASEB J 10:1031–1039
28. Lotan R (1995) Retinoids and apoptosis: implications for cancer chemoprevention and therapy. J Natl Cancer Inst 22:1655–1657
29. Hong WK, Lippman SM, Itri LM, Karp DD, Lee JS, Byers RM, Schantz SP, Kramer AM, Lotan R, Peters LJ, Dimery IW, Brown BW, Goepfert H (1993) Prevention of second primary tumors with isotretinoin in squamous cell carcinoma of the head and neck. N Engl J Med 323:795–801
30. Meyskens FL, Surwit E, Moon TE, Childers JM, Davis JR, Dorr RT, Johnson CS, Alberts DS (1994) Enhancement of regression of cervical intraepithelial neoplasia II (moderate dysplasia) with topically applied all-*trans*-retinoic acid: a randomized trial. J Natl Cancer Inst 86:539–543
31. Lu X-J, Fanjul A, Picard N, Pfahl M, Rungta D, Nared-Hood K, Carter B, Piedrafita J, Tang S, Fabbrizio E, Pfahl M (1997) Novel retinoid-related molecules as apoptosis inducers and effective inhibitors of human lung cancer cells in vivo. Nat Med 3:686–690

Subject Index

9784431702573